...ogram Your
Baby's Health

By Barbara Luke, Sc.D., M.P.H., R.D., and Tamara Eberlein:
When You're Expecting Twins, Triplets, or Quads

By Barbara Luke, Sc.D., M.P.H., R.D.:
*Good Bones: The Complete Guide to Building and
Maintaining the Healthiest Bones*
Multifetal Pregnancy: Care of the Pregnant Patient
(with Roger B. Newman, M.D.)

By Tamara Eberlein:
Sleep: How to Teach Your Child to Sleep Like a Baby
Whining: Tactics for Taming Demanding Behavior

Program Your Baby's Health

THE PREGNANCY DIET FOR YOUR CHILD'S LIFELONG WELL-BEING

*Barbara Luke, Sc.D., M.P.H., R.D.,
and Tamara Eberlein*

BALLANTINE BOOKS · NEW YORK

A Ballantine Book
Published by The Ballantine Publishing Group
Copyright © 2001 by Barbara Luke, Sc.D., M.P.H., R.D., and Tamara Eberlein

www.randomhouse.com/BB/

Library of Congress Cataloging-in-Publication Data
Luke, Barbara.
    Program your baby's health : the pregnancy diet for your child's lifelong
well-being / by Barbara Luke and Tamara Eberlein.—1st ed.
        p.   cm.
    ISBN 0-345-44199-0
    1. Pregnancy—Nutritional aspects.   2. Infants—Nutrition.   3. Prenatal
influences.   I. Eberlein, Tamara.   II. Title.
RG559.L846 2001
618.2'4—dc21   00-068067

Cover photo © VCG/FPG

Designed by Ann Gold

Manufactured in the United States of America

First Edition: April 2001

10   9   8   7   6   5   4   3   2   1

To my dear friend and colleague Mary L. Hediger,
who has spent her entire career making mothers
and their babies healthier.
—Barbara Luke

To my children, James, Samantha, and Jack Garvey,
with highest hopes for their bright futures.
—Tamara Eberlein

CONTENTS

We would like to give special thanks to the following individuals for their help in making this book a reality:

Kit Ward, Leslie Meredith and the staff at Ballantine Books, Mary Beth Voigt, Ruta Misiunas, and all the mothers who willingly shared their experiences during lengthy interviews.

Authors' Note:

The writing of this book was a joint effort. The term "I," as used in the text, refers to Dr. Barbara Luke and reflects her clinical expertise.

Program Your
Baby's Health

1 ✒ METABOLIC PROGRAMMING: THE NEW SCIENCE

Suppose a pregnant woman could take a pill that would program her unborn baby for a long and healthy life free of heart disease, hypertension, diabetes, cancer, asthma, allergies, and even obesity. Wouldn't every mother-to-be in the country clamor for a prescription?

Well, that miracle pill doesn't exist—but there is a prescription that can significantly boost your baby's odds of being born healthy and staying healthy for many decades. It's a prenatal regimen that lets an expectant mother "program" her unborn child for optimal growth, development, and resistance to disease from infancy through adulthood. Nearly all of the body's cells, systems, and organs may be positively and permanently affected by this regimen.

The key to this program lies in the cutting-edge research now under way in the scientific field known as *metabolic programming*. Evidence reveals that adult illnesses that have long been blamed on genetic influences or an unhealthy lifestyle may instead be the result of the uterine environment. In other words, *the nine short months of life in the womb may shape your baby's health as long as he or she lives.*

Prenatal nutrition is central to the health plan that can program your baby's health and metabolism. This plan involves no improbable menus and no hard-to-find, health-food-store-only fare. Instead, it's based on sound nutritional guidelines that incorporate real-people foods like pizza, cheeseburgers, chili, salads, and even ice cream into your diet. This is the plan I describe in *Program Your Baby's Health: The Pregnancy Diet for Your Child's Lifelong Well-being.*

As a medical school professor at the University of Michigan, public health nutritionist, epidemiologist, researcher, and mother myself, I am intimately familiar with both the science and the reality of maternal and pediatric nutrition. I have counseled thousands of pregnant women, and have helped generations of children to begin their lives healthy and strong.

For nearly three decades, metabolic programming has been the foundation of most of my research. It has also been the basis of my work as director of the University of Michigan Multiples Clinic, a highly successful program for women pregnant with twins, triplets, or quadruplets. At the clinic, we have designed a prenatal nutrition regimen that has resulted in hundreds of full-term, chubby-cheeked, healthy, beautiful babies. And this nutrition plan can do the same for your baby.

The Research Behind Metabolic Programming

Twenty-eight years ago, as a graduate student in nutrition, I read a shocking study that changed my life and the course of my career. The study detailed the findings of one thousand autopsies of stillborn children and analyzed their mothers' diets and weight gain during pregnancy[1]. It was a unique study because these babies had not died of any birth defect, but rather from complications during labor and delivery (tragedies that today are averted thanks to the routine use of electronic fetal monitoring). The study revealed that *when mothers were undernourished, their babies' organs were smaller and had fewer cells than normal.* Many different organs were adversely affected: the heart and lungs, the liver and kidneys, the thymus, and even the brain.

I wondered, had these babies lived, how these smaller organs and cellular deficits would have affected the children's health. Would the children have overcome the problems caused by these setbacks as they grew older, or would the ill effects have persisted throughout their lives? It seemed quite possible that inadequate lung development could lead to chronic asthma and respiratory problems; that an undersized liver might contribute to high cholesterol and cardiovascular disease in middle age; that poor growth of the kidneys could trigger hypertension; and that fewer thymus cells might translate into lifelong lowered immunity. These questions led a number of researchers, myself included, to examine the association between maternal nutrition and fetal, infant, and adult health.

Like pieces in a complicated puzzle, the answers to these questions nearly three decades ago have been put into place. All of the above concerns have proved to be valid: Smaller organs with fewer cells do set the stage for poor health later in life. Cellular deficits and other more subtle changes in the body's structure and function caused by inadequate prenatal nutrition support the concept that *many chronic diseases—including cardiovascular disease, hypertension, and diabetes—may originate before birth.*

The name for this new field of science has evolved as the body of research has grown. Originally referred to as the Barker hypothesis, then as the fetal origins theory, it is now known as metabolic programming. While this term is often used to describe the relationship between a poor uterine environment and long-term health problems, metabolic programming also includes a positive side: An optimal uterine environment can help to promote lifelong good health. I refer to this beneficial side of metabolic programming as positive programming.

EVIDENCE FROM AROUND THE WORLD

Evidence for the concept of metabolic programming comes from a variety of studies from across the globe. For instance:

• David Barker, a British epidemiologist, was one of the first researchers to provide direct evidence that certain adult-onset diseases could originate from growth retardation before birth[2]. His research team reported an important association between the risk of hypertension in adulthood and having been born weighing less than 5½ pounds.

• Further evidence for programming of adult hypertension in the womb was provided by the British National Study of Children[3]. Based on analysis of 5,362 individuals born in the United Kingdom in 1946 and followed to ages 43 or 44, this study demonstrated that adult blood pressure was significantly increased among individuals with low birthweight.

• The Dutch famine studies (based on the food blockage of the western Netherlands during World War II from October 1944 to May 1945) showed that women who were malnourished before they became pregnant experienced decreased fertility. Among children born to women who did get pregnant, there was an increase in birth defects of the spine and central nervous system, as well as an increase in mental illness in adulthood[4].

• The timing of the Dutch famine in relation to pregnancy was important, too. Women who were malnourished during the first two trimesters of their pregnancies had more premature births and more stillborn births, and their children experienced more obesity as adults[5]. Children born to women who were undernourished during the third trimester of pregnancy subsequently experienced less obesity as adults, but the girl babies who ultimately had children of their own were more likely to give birth to low-birthweight infants.

• Studies of pregnant women with diabetes indicate that episodes of starvation, even for short periods of time, can also have a negative effect on an unborn baby's developing nervous system. These children demonstrate lower IQ levels through nine years of age.

THE GOOD NEWS

I know that all of this can sound very scary. But please remember that there is a very positive side to metabolic programming: Just as poor nutrition during pregnancy can lead to long-term health problems for a child, optimal nutrition in pregnancy helps to reduce the risk of chronic disease and sets the stage for a child's long-term well-being. *By eating right when you're expecting, you can significantly boost your baby's chances of enjoying excellent lifelong health. It's that simple.*

Still skeptical? Let me explain more about how researchers have come to this conclusion. When investigating a disease, scientific researchers' first hint of its cause often comes from public health (or epidemiologic) studies. These studies look at clusters of cases that are linked to lifestyle or environmental factors. Recent examples include the connection between toxic shock syndrome and the use of Rely brand tampons, Legionnaires' disease and air-conditioning systems, and Kaposi's sarcoma and HIV. In investigating the causes of other medical conditions, scientists examine cellular, molecular, or genetic factors, and analyze how these may change in response to specific conditions.

Based on the strength of the research from hundreds of epidemiologic studies from around the world and combined with dramatic clinical evidence at the cellular level, the concept of metabolic programming has now become accepted as fact by scientists, researchers, and other health professionals in many fields. This accumulation of evidence for the validity of metabolic programming is one of the most exciting breakthroughs in the twentieth century, and is the basis for a highly effective new approach to the prevention of chronic disease in the twenty-first century.

Metabolic programming research provides powerful, compelling evidence that good nutrition before birth positively affects your baby's health. And these benefits endure not only through infancy and childhood, but throughout life, by permanently reducing your child's susceptibility to a variety of chronic diseases.

Why Growth Before Birth Is So Important

I tell my patients that pregnancy has a lot in common with gardening. You can't just throw seeds into soil, neglect to feed or water them, and still expect blue-ribbon roses. You have to nurture and nourish your potential showstoppers. So it's only logical that nutrition plays a major role in pregnancy as well, and that certain nutrients, or lack of them, at critical periods of development will have lasting significance. Your personal commitment to optimal nutrition will boost your baby's chances of lifelong well-being.

THE CRITICAL PERIOD

A critical period is when the cells of any developing organ or system are particularly sensitive to the environment inside the womb, and can be positively affected by certain nutrients. For instance, it's especially important for the mother to have enough folic acid in her diet immediately before and after conception (a critical period known as periconception) in order to ensure the baby's healthy spinal development. If folic acid is lacking during this period, the neural tube does not form properly and the baby will be born with spina bifida (an opening in the spine).

Development of other systems is similarly susceptible to the timing of nutrients delivered to the unborn baby via the mother's diet, particularly during periods of rapid growth and cell replication. During the first two months after conception (the embryonic period), the cells differentiate into the distinct organs and systems. From three months' gestation until birth (the fetal period) is the time of highest growth rate, when cells are multiplying. So the long-term positive programming effects of optimal nutrition and lifestyle behaviors (and the long-term negative programming effects of poor nutrition and other environmental factors) depend on the stage of pregnancy at which they occur.

Cells, tissues, and organs all develop in a marvelously ordered way from conception to maturity. Different organs and systems undergo periods of rapid cell division at different times. For instance:

- The critical period for the *heart* is early in pregnancy.
- For *kidney* development, the most crucial time is during late pregnancy.
- *Pancreatic cells* continue to differentiate even after birth, through the first months of infancy.
- *Lung* development is not complete until about two years of age.
- For the *brain and nervous system,* the critical period spans from early pregnancy through the first two years of life.

If the nutritional environment inside the womb is not ideal during any critical period, the baby's body adapts to what is available. Although this adaptation improves its chances for immediate survival, the cost to the child's health may become apparent only years later. The child's increased risk for developing certain chronic diseases may even remain dormant for decades until triggered by other negative factors or lifestyle choices later on, such as obesity or smoking.

For all these reasons, your baby needs the best nutrition you can provide at each stage of pregnancy and into childhood in order to be healthy and strong. In this way you help to ensure that your child grows and develops as wonderfully as nature intended.

Using Metabolic Programming to the Best Advantage

The period from preconception through the first few years of life provides an extraordinary window of opportunity to lay a strong foundation for your child's optimal health. As an expectant mother who follows the positive programming plan outlined in this book, you will be empowered to protect your child's future health in a multitude of ways. You'll learn the following things:

Appropriate weight gain is a vital safeguard for future health.
• When a pregnant woman is careful to gain enough weight, her child receives added protection against heart disease. That's because an undernourished fetus shunts blood to its brain at the expense of the organs of the abdomen. As a consequence, the baby's liver ends up being smaller than normal, and therefore less efficient at clearing cholesterol from the bloodstream. This can contribute to heart disease in adulthood.
• Sufficient weight gain also guards against a diabetic future. When an expectant mother eats too little, her fetus develops a "thrifty metabolism" that hoards every available calorie. Later, during childhood and adulthood, when this metabolism is challenged by an abundance of food, the individual is much more likely to become obese and to develop diabetes.

Certain nutrients help prevent specific, predictable problems.
• A pregnancy diet rich in protein may help your child avoid hypertension down the road. Insufficient protein prevents an enzyme in the placenta from deactivating harmful hormones such as cortisol. When this occurs, the baby's set point for blood pressure may be permanently raised.
• Adequate dietary protein also guards against diabetes. When protein is lacking, the pancreas develops fewer blood vessels in the

cells that produce insulin, thereby setting the stage for the later development of diabetes.

• With adequate dietary magnesium and omega-3 fatty acids, blood flow to the placenta is protected. When the supply of these nutrients is insufficient, the consequences include damage to the placental blood vessels, an increased risk of premature labor, and other problems.

• Magnesium also helps to boost immunity and to protect the fetus's developing nervous system.

• A diet rich in essential fatty acids, like omega-3, aids neurological development and boosts intelligence.

• Essential fatty acids are also key to the development of normal vision.

• An iron rich diet promotes proper growth of the placenta, the vital organ responsible for transmitting nutrients and oxygen to your unborn baby. A healthy placenta maximizes the genetic potential for your baby to thrive.

When (not just what) a woman eats is crucial, too.

• Adequate weight gain early in pregnancy guards against nervous system defects and perhaps schizophrenia. (That's one reason why morning sickness should be taken far more seriously than it generally is, a topic discussed at length in Chapter 5.)

• Proper nourishment during the first trimester of pregnancy decreases the risk that your child will become obese later in life. When maternal nutrition is inadequate early in pregnancy, the appetite-control centers in the unborn baby's brain may be permanently altered, leading to an urge to overeat in later life.

• The majority of kidney growth occurs during the last three months of pregnancy. Proper nutrition at this stage can help protect against chronic kidney problems as well as hypertension.

• The third trimester is an important time of growth for the lungs. Poor nutrition can reduce lung size, leading to greater susceptibility to respiratory tract infections, chronic bronchitis, and sensitivity to environmental pollutants in childhood and beyond.

Certain pregnancies involve special metabolic programming concerns.

• Boys are more vulnerable to the negative effects of under-nutrition because they have a more rapid growth pattern. If pre-natal testing reveals that you are carrying a boy, you can take extra steps to assure that your diet is optimal.

• Twin and supertwin pregnancies (triplets, quadruplets, and more) involve far greater nutritional needs—even more than many obstetricians may realize. Multiple-birth babies are pro-tected when an expectant mother makes wise dietary and lifestyle choices.

• A woman who has undergone infertility treatments is more likely to have depleted nutrient stores and to suffer from morning sickness. If you are a former infertility patient, this prenatal pro-gram can give you the specific advice you need in order to have the healthiest child possible.

Metabolic programming doesn't end with childbirth.

• Many bodily systems are still vulnerable to the effects of metabolic programming during the first two years after birth, or even into adolescence. Proper nourishment during infancy and childhood can reduce the risk of a multitude of health problems later in life, including cardiovascular disease, the number-one killer of Americans.

• Lung development is not complete until the second or third year after birth. Careful avoidance of environmental pollutants such as cigarette smoke during infancy and toddlerhood can im-prove lung health, particularly among children who were born small. Otherwise, the child is at increased risk for respiratory tract infections and chronic bronchitis, and this risk often lasts through adulthood.

• Pancreatic cells continue to differentiate during infancy. Because a child's diet affects the way his or her tissues respond to insulin, proper nutrition decreases his risk for diabetes.

• Good nutrition during infancy, childhood, and the teen years helps to ensure a lowered risk for many chronic diseases. Chapters 8 and 9 provide the information you need to enhance the positive effects of metabolic programming even after your child is born.

Some of my patients get tired of hearing about nutrition and weight gain and what they should eat. One woman even ribbed me for being so adamant about the importance of diet. But she did stick with the program, and her babies were born big and healthy. A few days after she delivered, she came to me and said, "I just passed by the neonatal intensive care unit and saw all these babies who were so much smaller than my daughters. I finally understood why you kept on my case about eating right. Thank you for being my babies' nutrition advocate."

Please let me be an advocate for your baby, too. My instructions won't be difficult to follow, I promise. This book translates the concept of metabolic programming into a practical, easy-to-understand, day-to-day nutrition and lifestyle program. Follow the guidelines, and you'll be offering your child the very best opportunity to be born healthy and to stay healthy for many decades to come.

2 ℐ❧ YOUR UNBORN BABY'S NUTRITIONAL NEEDS

Prenatal nutrition is at the heart of metabolic programming. So keep in mind this one simple goal: You want to create an optimal nutritional environment for your unborn baby so that he or she can grow and develop in the very best ways possible. This is achieved by eating the right kinds of foods, in the right amounts, at the right time of day, throughout your pregnancy. As a consequence, you greatly reduce your child's risk of developing any of a number of chronic diseases associated with poor prenatal nutrition.

If you are already pregnant, congratulations! The majority of the nutrition information in this chapter can benefit you and your unborn baby, whether you conceived just a few days ago or are already well into your pregnancy. Please read it carefully before moving on to the later chapters, where we'll discuss issues specific to each of the three trimesters of pregnancy. In this way, you help to ensure that your unborn baby will reap the benefits of positive programming.

If you're reading this book in anticipation of becoming pregnant, know that the effects of metabolic programming begin from the moment of conception, so you want your body to be as prepared as possible for that moment. Through the foods you eat, you can do a great deal in the weeks and months before you conceive, to set the stage for a healthy pregnancy. As you read this chapter, pay special attention to the end of each section, where you'll find subheads that begin, "If you're planning to get pregnant . . ." By following the advice meant specifically for women who have not yet conceived, you will set the stage for having a pregnancy in which you will feel your best and your baby will thrive.

Your Personal Nutritional Status

You can't fool Mother Nature: Nutrition is the foundation for good health. In order to feel and look your best, a healthful diet must be a regular part of your daily routine. Diet is even more important during pregnancy for two reasons. First, pregnancy places additional physical and emotional demands on a woman, and these demands are met primarily through appropriate nutrition. Second, and most important in terms of metabolic programming, an unborn baby's ability to grow is determined mainly by the mother's supply of nutrients. Almost all of the nourishment your unborn baby receives comes from what you eat.

Your ability to nourish your unborn baby is also affected by the circumstances of your own fetal life—in other words, by how well nourished you yourself were before birth. *Adverse nutritional effects from one generation can negatively affect the next generation.* Health professionals have noted that among immigrants to the United States the benefits of improved nutrition are often not seen until the second generation. Similarly, studies have shown that women who suffered from malnutrition during the first half of their pregnancies often had daughters with a normal birthweight, yet a generation later these daughters' babies showed an increased incidence of growth restriction.

TABLE 2-1. TOP 25 ALL-STAR FOODS

Food Group	Food	Nutritional Benefits
Dairy	Yogurt	Easily digested, high-quality protein, low glycemic-index carbohydrate, calcium, magnesium, phosphorus, zinc, immunologic qualities, riboflavin, and vitamins B_{12} and D
	Skim milk	High-quality protein, nonfat, low glycemic-index carbohydrate, calcium, iodine, magnesium, phosphorus, potassium, vitamins A, D, B_{12}, and riboflavin
	Cheese	High-quality protein and calcium
Protein	Coldwater fish	High-quality protein, vitamins A and B_{12}, niacin, biotin, calcium, riboflavin, and omega-3 essential fatty acids
	Shellfish	High-quality protein, lowfat, calcium, copper, iodine, manganese, and vitamin D
	Eggs	High-quality protein, chromium, phosphorus, zinc, vitamins A, B_6, and D, and biotin
	Lean beef	High-quality protein, iron, chromium, selenium, zinc, thiamin, pantothenic acid, pyridoxine, and vitamin B_{12}
	Lean pork	High-quality protein, iron, chromium, thiamin, pantothenic acid, and vitamin B_{12}
	Lean poultry	High-quality protein, iron, chromium, selenium, zinc, thiamin, pantothenic acid, pyridoxine, and vitamin B_{12}
	Tofu	Protein, lowfat, fiber, vitamin A, thiamin, folic acid, calcium, zinc, and anticancer phytonutrients

Category	Food	Nutrients
Legumes	Beans, peas, lentils, chickpeas	Protein, lowfat, fiber, low glycemic index carbohydrate, folic acid, thiamin, pyridoxine, calcium, copper, iron, and zinc
Nuts	Peanuts, cashews, walnuts	Protein, fiber, copper, magnesium, manganese, zinc, pyridoxine, and biotin
Vegetables	Asparagus	Fiber, vitamins A, C, and E, riboflavin, folic acid, thiamin, copper, magnesium, and potassium
	Broccoli	Fiber, vitamins A, C, K, riboflavin, folic acid, calcium, chromium, magnesium, and manganese
	Cabbage	Fiber, vitamins A, C, K, riboflavin, and folic acid
	Pumpkin	Fiber, vitamins A and C, and chromium
	Spinach	Calcium, chromium, iron, magnesium, manganese, potassium, vitamins A, C, K, riboflavin, and folic acid
	Sweet potatoes, yams	Fiber, vitamin A, low glycemic index carbohydrate, and chromium
	Tomatoes	Vitamins A and C and carotenoids, especially lycopene and lutein
Fruits	Apples	Fiber, chromium, and low glycemic-index carbohydrate
	Avocados	Fiber, B vitamins, vitamins A and E, copper, magnesium, potassium, and pyridoxine
	Cherries	Low glycemic-index carbohydrate, and vitamins A and C
	Oranges	Fiber, low glycemic-index carbohydrate, vitamins A and C, and folic acid
Grains	Oatmeal	Protein, fiber, low glycemic-index carbohydrate, iron, magnesium, manganese, selenium, and zinc
	Wheat germ	Protein, fiber, lowfat, vitamin E, thiamin, folic acid, magnesium, phosphorus, and zinc

Furthermore, your nutritional history from childhood, adolescence, and adulthood plays a role in your baby's development. For certain nutrients, an unborn baby draws on the mother's own reserves. When those nutrient reserves are deficient, the baby's development is compromised. You can't change your nutritional history. Nonetheless, you can greatly improve the odds of good health for your unborn baby and for yourself by taking steps now to improve your nutritional status. And you'll also be improving the health of your future grandchildren.

DON'T WORRY, IT'S EASY

Are you worried that it seems like a lot of work to figure out what and when and how much you should eat? Well, take heart—I've done all this work for you. Look at the menus and meal plans at the end of each chapter, as well as the recipes in the back of the book. They take the guesswork out of eating right when you're expecting so you can concentrate on the joys of being pregnant.

◄ *If you're planning to get pregnant,* understand that your partner's nutritional status affects your ability to get pregnant. For instance, men whose diets are deficient in zinc or vitamin C can become infertile[1]. Severe nutritional deficiencies can cause a decrease in sperm count and quality, and a weight loss greater than 25 percent of normal body weight can cause sperm production to cease entirely[2]. So, as you improve your diet in preparation for pregnancy, encourage the future father to eat right, too.

THE TOP 25 FOOD ALL-STARS

Here's a simple way to improve your diet, starting today: Eat more of what I call the Top 25 Food All-Stars. In compiling this list, my main criteria included high nutrient content, flavor, and versatility as an ingredient in recipes. These foods are shown in Table 2-1.

I've also featured these All-Stars in the recipes at the back of this book. Each recipe is rated in two ways: (1) with a spoon rating for the number of Top 25 Food All-Stars included in the recipe; (2) and with a star rating indicating the number of nutrients the recipe provides, per serving, at a level of 20 percent or more of the Daily Recommended Intake for adults.

For most people, a diet that is defined in terms of grams and milligrams of food means next to nothing. People want to read recommendations that give specific numbers of servings—like how many pieces of chicken, slices of cheese, and glasses of milk to eat daily. So that's exactly what I've done. Table 2-2 tells you how many servings of real foods to eat each day. The recommendations are further divided to reflect the specific dietary needs of four different types of women:

- women who are planning to get pregnant
- women in the first trimester of pregnancy
- women in the second or third trimester of pregnancy
- nursing mothers

In using Table 2-2, please pay attention to the section called Portion Size, which gives examples of typical serving sizes for each category of food. For instance, my recommendation to get six daily servings of meat or meat equivalents (such as eggs, peanut butter, and beans) during pregnancy means you need *six ounces* of meat total—not six porterhouse steaks!

◀ *If you're planning to get pregnant,* you should start right now to establish good eating habits. Our daily diet should include:

- at least six to eight servings of fruits and vegetables
- three servings of dairy foods
- four to six servings of meat or meat equivalents
- six to eight servings of breads and grains
- two to three servings of oils or nuts

TABLE 2-2. MENU GUIDELINES FOR BEFORE, DURING, AND AFTER PREGNANCY

Food	Portion Size	Nonpregnant	Pregnant 1ST TRIMESTER	Pregnant 2ND & 3RD TRIMESTERS	Breastfeeding
Dairy	8 oz. skim or lowfat milk 8 oz. yogurt 1/4 cup cottage cheese 1 oz. hard cheese	3	4	6	8
Meat, fish, or poultry Cooked beans Cooked lentils	1 oz. 1 cup 1/2 cup	4–6	6	6	6
Eggs	1 fresh	0–1	0–1	1	1
Vegetables	1/2 cup cooked or 1 cup fresh	3–4	4	4	4
Fruits	1/2 cup or 1 whole, fresh	3–4	4	4	4
Breads Cereals Pasta, rice, potatoes	1 oz., 1 slice 3/4 cup 1/2 cup cooked	6–8	8	8	8
Fats, oils, and nuts	1 tbsp. oil 1 pat butter 1 oz. nuts	2–3	4	5	5

- an adequate intake of folic acid
- enough iron-rich foods to boost your iron stores

A New Way to Think About Food

In today's fast-paced environment, many women see food primarily as a quick source of energy, something to grab on the fly and eat on the go. For others, food is a friend to turn to, with the "comfort factor" of chocolate or potato chips taking precedence over nutritional quality. And for some women, food is an enemy to avoid in an ongoing battle for a slimmer figure.

However, when you're pregnant or trying to get pregnant you need to think of food in a whole new way—not as fuel, friend, or foe, but as an ally. The food you eat is the most important factor in determining how well your unborn baby grows and develops. And that's fortunate, *because your diet is one aspect of your pregnancy over which you have complete control*

So learn to listen your body. It's telling you to eat well and often, and to choose foods that are nutrient rich.

WHY YOU SHOULD EAT MORE OFTEN

You're probably not surprised to be told to eat well, but you may wonder why I want you to eat often—at least every three hours. The central issue is blood glucose control, which means maintaining an appropriate blood sugar level.

This is vital because your unborn baby's nervous system needs a constant supply of glucose in order to develop properly. When you skip meals or go too long without a snack, your blood sugar level drops and your baby is deprived of the glucose he or she needs. Fasting is particularly dangerous because it leads to extremely low blood sugar, or hypoglycemia, which can trigger preterm labor.

Poor blood glucose control also affects how you feel. For instance, suppose you haven't eaten in five or six hours. Your blood sugar is low, so you feel fatigued and irritable. You grab a jelly doughnut, and soon your blood sugar soars, leaving you hyper and jittery. Your pancreas responds by producing high levels of insulin, which causes your blood sugar level to drop back down even lower than it was before you ate the doughnut. Soon, you're more lethargic and moody than before—a victim of a vicious cycle. Plus, there's an unhealthy long-term consequence: The flood of insulin triggers your body to increase its storage of body fat.

Clearly, such swings in blood glucose are not good for you or your baby. Yet if you are like many women, they are a daily occurrence, the result of an eating schedule gone awry—when your breakfast is a cup of coffee and your lunch is fast (or fast food), the munchies hit you by midafternoon, so dinnertime finds you famished, and you finish with a big sweet snack late at night. If this sounds like you, your caloric distribution is probably 5 percent for breakfast, 20 percent for lunch, 20–25 percent for the midafternoon snack, 30–35 percent for dinner, and 15–25 percent for a bedtime snack.

To keep blood glucose within the normal range, you should divide your day's calories as follows:

Meal	Percent of Total Calories	Calories Per Meal or Snack
Breakfast	15–20	375–500
Midmorning snack	5–10	125–250
Lunch	30	750
Midafternoon snack	5–10	125–250
Dinner	30	750
Evening snack	5–10	125–250

In addition, you should *include protein with every meal or snack.* Because protein is digested slowly, it allows sugar to enter your bloodstream at a more even rate. Fiber has the same stabilizing effect on blood sugar because it also slows digestion. *Avoid foods high in simple sugars*—candy, pastries, regular soft drinks, jellies, and jams—particularly on an empty stomach. These foods wreak havoc with your blood glucose level because they are digested quickly.

You may be surprised to learn that this eating schedule and food-choice advice are basically the same as the ones recommended for individuals with diabetes. It's been said, "If you want to live a long and healthy life, get a chronic disease and take care of it." Those words of wisdom are pretty much on the mark. The healthiest way to eat before, during, and after pregnancy is as if you have diabetes.

In my practice of counseling women pregnant with twins, triplets, or quadruplets, I put everyone on a diabetic diet the minute they walk through my office door. And I recommend the same for you, whether you're expecting one baby or more than one. For any pregnant woman, maintaining blood glucose within a healthy range should be a top priority, twenty-four hours a day, seven days a week.

Here are additional strategies for accomplishing that goal:

- Eat at least every three hours.
- Eat at around the same time every day, and keep your meals about the same size from day to day.
- In every snack or meal, include a protein food such as milk, cheese, cottage cheese, yogurt, meat, fish, poultry, or nuts.
- Get plenty of fiber by including foods such as bran and whole-grain cereals, fruits, and vegetables.
- Avoid sugary treats and limit your use of artificial sweeteners. Satisfy your sweet tooth with fresh or dried fruits.
- Fruit is preferable to fruit juice, because fruit's extra fiber means it is digested more slowly. Do not eat fruit or drink fruit juice on an empty stomach.

- Breads digest quickly, so they too should not be eaten on an empty stomach. At breakfast, limit bread to one slice, preferably whole-wheat, rye, or high-fiber.

An added benefit in following these dietary guidelines is that you will gain weight in a healthy pattern, which aids your baby's development in numerous ways. Plus, by the end of your pregnancy, you will not have lost muscle, nor put on too much additional body fat. You will be able to return to your prepregnancy weight and shape much more quickly—which is healthy for your body as well as uplifting for your spirits.

Nutrition Made Simple

When health professionals like me speak about nutrition, we are referring to the six groups of essential nutrients found in foods: *proteins, carbohydrates, and fats* (the macronutrients); *vitamins and minerals* (the micronutrients); and *water.* Each one of these plays a vital role in your unborn baby's development.

To get the maximum nutritional benefit from the foods you eat when you're pregnant, remember these three key points:

- Get 20 to 25 percent of your day's calories from protein, 40 to 50 percent from carbohydrates, and 30 to 40 percent from fats.
- Eat a variety of foods.
- Choose foods that are fresh or have been minimally processed— in other words, foods that are as close to their original state as possible.

THE PROTEINS
Proteins are the body's basic building blocks, and as such, they are the most vital nutrient for your baby's growth. Babies who are well

grown at birth, even if they are born prematurely, have fewer illnesses and recover from them more quickly than babies with poor prenatal growth.

Proteins are made up of amino acids—structural units that are essential for building and repairing tissue, and for the formation of blood, bones, and the brain. Amino acids are also important components of enzymes, hormones, and the antibodies that are part of the immune system.

Some of the amino acids in protein cannot be made by our own bodies. These are called the *essential amino acids*, and they must be included in the diet. Protein foods that contain all essential amino acids (called complete proteins) include:

- meat
- fish
- poultry
- eggs
- dairy products such as milk and cheese

If you are a vegetarian, you must be especially careful to combine foods properly so that you get all the essential amino acids in your meals. Combinations that achieve this goal include:

- cereal with milk
- macaroni and cheese
- peanut butter with whole-grain bread
- rice with beans

Once you become pregnant, you need extra protein. This protein is used to build the placenta; to allow for increases in breast tissue, uterine tissue, and blood volume; and to promote your baby's growth. I'm not recommending that you follow a high-protein diet; it's better to follow a *quality-protein* diet. Remember, while you should get 20 to 25 percent of your daily calories from protein, a higher percentage—around 40 to 50 percent of the day's calories—should come from carbohydrates.

Many popular weight-reducing diets promote high-protein regimens that exclude carbohydrates. Yet without the help of carbohydrates, the body inefficiently burns protein and fat, and excretes the by-products of this metabolism (called *ketones*) in the urine. While the presence of ketones in the urine (called *ketonuria*) is usually not harmful to adults, it is very harmful to the developing baby because carbohydrates are the only source of energy the unborn baby can use. When you don't get enough carbohydrates and calories, your body switches over to burning fats and proteins, a process known as *accelerated starvation*. This can be damaging to your baby's developing nervous system. In clinical studies, ketonuria and accelerated starvation during pregnancy have been linked to lower IQs in children.

How much protein do you need?
About 20 to 25 percent of your daily calories should come from protein. If you're underweight, aim for the high end of the range shown below; if you're overweight, stick to the low end of the range:

- Get 100 to 125 grams of protein per day before you get pregnant.
- Get 110 to 138 grams of protein per day during the first trimester.
- Get 125 to 156 grams of protein per day during the second and third trimesters.
- Get 135 to 169 grams of protein per day during breastfeeding.

THE CARBOHYDRATES
Carbohydrates are the only energy source for your unborn baby's developing nervous system. They also provide the primary energy

source for adults. This is why the greatest percentage of calories in your daily diet should come from carbohydrates.

Sometimes called sugars, carbohydrates come in two forms: simple (or refined) and complex (or starches). The simple sugar fructose is found in fruits and fruit juices, honey, and refined sugar; the simple sugar galactose is found in milk and dairy products. Complex carbohydrates include grains, breads, cereals, pasta, and certain vegetables. The majority of your carbohydrate calories should come from carbohydrates with fiber, such as whole-grain breads and cereals, and from fruits and vegetables, rather than from refined sugars.

Dietary Fiber

The nondigestible source of carbohydrate found in all plant foods (fruits, vegetables, grains, nuts, and seeds) is called dietary fiber. There are two types of dietary fiber: insoluble and soluble. The insoluble fiber found in the cell walls of all plant foods is called cellulose. Soluble fiber is also found in the cell walls of plants, and is concentrated in the skins and rinds of fruits and vegetables. During digestion, soluble fiber dissolves to form a soft gel.

Mounting scientific evidence links the consumption of dietary fiber with reductions in heart disease, cancer, and diabetes. By absorbing water as it passes through the digestive tract, insoluble fiber helps to prevent constipation and perhaps reduces the risk of colon cancer. Fiber also stabilizes blood sugar levels by slowing the rate at which carbohydrates enter the bloodstream. The downside of fiber from grain foods (grains, cereals, breads, pasta, and rice) is that it binds with minerals, specifically calcium, and prevents their absorption. The fiber in fruits and vegetables, however, has no such disadvantage.

The American Heart Association, the National Cancer Institute, and the National Institutes of Health all recommend consuming *20 to 35 grams of dietary fiber daily*. The most recent revision of the U.S. Department of Agriculture (USDA) Dietary

TABLE 2-3. DIETARY SOURCES OF FIBER

Food		Amount	Total Carbohydrates (grams)	Dietary Fiber (grams)	Percent of Carbohydrates as Dietary Fiber*
Breads and cereals	Fiber 1 (General Mills)	1 oz. (½ c)	24.0	13.0	54%
	All-Bran (Kellogg's)	1 oz. (½ c)	24.0	10.0	42%
	Bran Buds (Kellogg's)	1 oz. (½ c)	22.0	8.0	36%
	Raisin Bran	1 cup	46.0	8.0	17%
	Bran Chex (Ralston Purina)	1 oz. (⅔ c)	23.0	6.1	27%
	Cracklin' Oat Bran (Kellogg's)	¾ cup	35.0	6.0	17%
	Kellogg's Complete	¾ cup	23.0	5.0	22%
	Shredded wheat	2 biscuits	38.0	5.0	13%
	Weetabix	2 biscuits	28.0	5.0	19%
	Regular Oatmeal (Quaker Oats)	½ cup dry	27.0	4.0	15%
	Instant Oatmeal (Quaker Oats)	1 packet	19.9	3.0	15%
	Wheaties (General Mills)	1 oz. (1 c)	24.0	3.0	13%
	Ry Krisp Sesame	2 crackers	11.0	3.0	27%
	Multi-Grain Cheerios (General Mills)	1 cup	24.0	3.0	13%
	Cheerios (General Mills)	1 cup	22.0	3.0	14%
	Total Whole Grain (General Mills)	¾ cup	23.0	3.0	13%
	Fiber-Plus Crispbread (Wasa)	1 slice	5.0	2.8	56%
	Grape-Nuts (Post)	1 oz. (¼ c)	23.1	2.6	11%
	Crispbread (Wasa) Sesame Rye	1 slice	4.0	2.4	60%
	Life (Quaker Oats)	¾ cup	25.0	2.0	8%
	Wheat germ	2 tbsp.	6.0	2.0	33%
	Natural whole wheat bread (Brownberry)	1 slice	16.9	2.3	14%
	Whole wheat bread (Roman meal)	1 slice	12.9	1.6	12%

	Food	Serving		%
	Jewish rye with seeds (Arnold)	1 slice	14.6	1.3	9%
	Kix (General Mills)	1⅓ cups	26.0	1.0	4%
	Corn Flakes (Kellogg's)	1 cup	24.0	1.0	4%
	Toasted Wheat Crispbread (Wasa)	1 slice	9.0	1.0	11%
	Cap'n Krunch	¾ cup	23.0	1.0	4%
	Special K (Kellogg's)	1 cup	23.0	1.0	4%
	White bread	1 slice	11.3	0.8	7%
	Oatmeal bread	1 slice	13.0	0.6	5%
	Raisin bread	1 slice	13.2	0.6	5%
	Rice Krispies (Kellogg's)	1¼ cups	29.0	0.0	0%
Nuts and nut foods	Coconut, dried and sweetened	⅓ cup	10.4	3.7	36%
	Almonds, dry roasted	1 oz.	5.4	3.1	57%
	Pistachios	1 oz.	7.1	3.0	42%
	Mixed nuts	1 oz.	6.1	2.5	41%
	Peanuts, dry roasted	1 oz.	6.0	2.2	37%
	Peanut butter	2 tbsp.	6.6	2.0	30%
	Pecans	1 oz.	5.2	1.8	35%
	Cashews	1 oz.	8.1	1.7	21%
	Walnuts	1 oz.	5.2	1.3	25%
Fruits	Prunes, dried	10	52.7	6.0	11%
	Raspberries	1 cup	14.2	5.8	41%
	Raisins	⅔ cup	79.1	5.3	7%
	Figs	5 medium	28.0	5.0	18%
	Avocados	1 medium	12.0	4.7	39%
	Dates	10 medium	61.0	4.2	7%
	Pear	1 medium	25.1	4.3	17%
	Strawberries	1 cup	10.5	3.9	37%
	Blueberries	1 cup	20.5	3.3	16%
	Apples	1 medium	21.1	3.0	14%

Food	Amount	Total Carbohydrates (grams)	Dietary Fiber (grams)	Percent of Carbohydrates as Dietary Fiber*
Oranges	1 medium	14.4	2.9	20%
Mango	1 medium	35.2	2.2	6%
Pineapple	1 cup	19.2	1.9	10%
Bananas	1 medium	26.7	1.8	7%
Apricots	3 medium	11.8	1.4	12%
Peaches	1 medium	9.7	1.4	14%
Cantaloupe	1 cup	13.4	1.3	10%
Cherries, fresh	10	11.3	1.1	10%
Vegetables				
Baked beans (Bush's Best)	½ cup	29.0	7.0	24%
Refried beans	½ cup	20.0	6.0	30%
Pumpkin, canned	½ cup	10.1	3.8	38%
Three-bean salad	½ cup	22.6	3.2	14%
Corn, boiled	½ cup	20.6	3.0	15%
Chickpeas (garbanzo beans)	½ cup	22.5	2.9	13%
Squash, baked	½ cup	8.9	2.9	33%
Green peas, cooked	½ cup	10.7	2.9	27%
Broccoli, cooked	½ cup	4.0	2.0	50%
Red cabbage, cooked	½ cup	3.5	1.8	51%
Carrots, cooked	½ cup	8.2	1.5	18%
Cauliflower, cooked	½ cup	2.9	1.4	48%
Corn, canned	½ cup	15.2	1.1	7%
Green beans, cooked	½ cup	4.9	1.1	22%

*Italic type indicates that 20% or more of a food's carbohydrate content is in the form of dietary fiber.

Guidelines for Americans (graphically presented as the Food Guide Pyramid) recommends that adults get two to four servings per day of fruits, three to five servings per day of vegetables, and six to eleven servings per day of grain foods. Yet recent national surveys indicate that only one out of four Americans eats this much fruit, only one in eight meets the recommendation for vegetables, and fewer than half get sufficient grains.

How can you tell if you're getting enough fiber? Best sources include bran and whole-grain cereals, fresh and dried fruits, and raw vegetables. For a more complete list, refer to Table 2-3. (In this table, foods are divided into categories. Within each category, items are listed in order of fiber content, from the highest fiber to the lowest.)

As you can see from Table 2-3, you can't rely on the "crunch factor" to identify high-fiber foods. For instance, saltine crackers have no fiber, and a stalk of celery has a meager one-half of a gram. Many breakfast cereals and granola bars are likewise low in dietary fiber, yet high in sugars and fats. On the other hand, creamy smooth pumpkin contains a whopping 5 grams of fiber per half-cup serving, while canned sweet peas provide 4 grams per half cup.

Recent changes in food labeling regulations have made it easier to identify sources of dietary fiber. For a food to be labeled a good source of fiber, it must contain at least 2.5 to 4.9 grams of fiber per serving. To be labeled high fiber, it must contain 5 grams or more per serving.

The Best Carbohydrates for Your Unborn Baby

Clearly, all carbohydrates are not created equal. You want your carbohydrate foods to be high in fiber and low in glucose.

One way of determining the best foods for you to eat in general, as well as during your pregnancy, is to refer to the *glycemic index*. This is a measure of the rate of entry of carbohydrates into the bloodstream, which affects your blood sugar level after a meal.

As we discussed before, you want to maintain a stable level of blood sugar. Foods that enter the bloodstream too rapidly can undermine this goal. Several factors influence a food's glycemic index:

- the structure of the carbohydrates that are present
- the soluble and insoluble fiber content
- the fat content

All simple sugars (glucose, galactose, and fructose) are rapidly absorbed by the liver, but only glucose is directly released into the bloodstream. This explains why glucose-rich foods like pasta, cereals, and breads have the highest glycemic index, while the most fructose-rich fruits and vegetables, and galactose-rich dairy products, have the lowest glycemic index. Insoluble fiber also slows down the rate of entry of carbohydrate into the bloodstream, thereby lowering a food's glycemic index.

Most fruits and fiber-rich vegetables are low-glycemic foods, while all grains, starches, and pastas are high-glycemic carbohydrates. Processed foods, such as canned vegetables and fruit juices, are reduced in fiber content and therefore have a higher glycemic index. Table 2-4 provides a list of various foods and their glycemic index.

TABLE 2-4. THE GLYCEMIC INDEX OF COMMON FOODS

GLYCEMIC INDEX GREATER THAN OR EQUAL TO 100%

Breads, grains, and cereals

Bagels	Corn Flakes cereal
Bread stuffing	Crispix cereal
Cheerios cereal	French bread
Corn Chex cereal	Golden Grahams cereal
Corn chips	Puffed Rice cereal

Puffed wheat cereal
Rice Chex cereal
Rice Krispies cereal
Total cereal
White bread

Fruits and vegetables
Baked potatoes
Carrots
Instant rice
Parsnips
Watermelon

GLYCEMIC INDEX BETWEEN 80 AND 100%

Breads, grains, and cereals

Bran Chex cereal
Brown rice
Cream of Wheat cereal
Grape Nuts cereal
Hamburger bun
Instant mashed potatoes
Life cereal
Macaroni and cheese
Oat bran
Rolled oats
Ry-Krisp crackers

Shredded wheat
White rice
Whole-wheat bread

Fruits and vegetables
Apricots
Mango
Papaya
Pineapple
Raisins

GLYCEMIC INDEX BETWEEN 50 AND 80%

Breads, grains, and cereals

Pasta
All-Bran cereal
Pumpernickel bread
Special K cereal
Sweet corn, canned

Fruits and vegetables
Baked beans
Bananas
Garbanzo beans

Grapes
Kidney beans
Navy beans
Oranges
Orange juice
Peas
Pinto beans
Popcorn
Sweet potatoes
Yams

GLYCEMIC INDEX BETWEEN 30 AND 50%

Breads, grains, and cereals

Barley
Oatmeal (slow-cooking)
Whole-grain rye bread

Fruits and vegetables
Apples
Apple juice
Applesauce
Apricots (dried)
Black-eyed peas
Grapefruit

Kidney beans (dried)
Lentils
Lima beans
Peaches
Pears
Tomato soup

Dairy products
Ice cream
Milk
Yogurt

GLYCEMIC INDEX OF 30% OR LESS

Cherries
Peanuts
Peas

Plums
Soybeans

Your goal is to limit your consumption of foods with a glycemic index greater than 80 percent. When you do consume high-glycemic foods, eat them in combination with a protein or high-fiber food. This helps you to maintain a stable blood sugar level and promotes the positive programming of your baby's nervous system.

How Much Carbohydrate Do You Need?

About 40–50% of your daily calories should come from carbohydrates. If you're underweight, aim for the high end of the range shown below; if you're overweight, stick to the low end of the range:

- Get 200 to 250 grams of carbohydrate per day before you get pregnant.
- Get 220 to 275 grams of carbohydrate per day during the first trimester.
- Get 250 to 312 grams of carbohydrate per day during the second and third trimesters.
- Get 270 to 338 grams of carbohydrate per day during breast-feeding.

THE FATS

You may be accustomed to thinking of all fats as something to be scrupulously avoided in your quest for good health and a trim figure. But your unborn baby needs certain types of fats for proper neurologic development, for good vision, and to reduce the risk of premature birth.

Ounce for ounce, fat is the most concentrated source of energy in our diets. It provides nine calories per gram—more than twice as much as protein or carbohydrates. Although all fats have an equivalent caloric content, there are different types of fats—and while some do indeed harm your health, others are necessary for good health.

Certain types of fat are termed *essential* because our bodies cannot make them, and so we must get them from dietary sources. These essential fats include the *omega-3 fatty acids* and the *omega-6 fatty acids*. Both of these form biological compounds in the body that affect functions such as blood pressure, blood clotting, and the immune response. In addition, the omega-3 fatty acids reduce the risk of cardiovascular disease by improving the body's ability to synthesize and get rid of harmful lipoproteins. They also may provide some protection against breast cancer.

Essential fatty acids are also vital to the well-being of your unborn baby. For instance, the omega-3s are the type of fat that promotes good development of your baby's vision and nervous system. Omega-3s also appear to inhibit the synthesis of prosta-glandin, a substance that initiates preterm labor. This is why your diet must include adequate amounts of the "good fats" through-out your pregnancy, and most particularly during the third tri-mester and while breastfeeding. Pregnant women who develop a condition called gestational diabetes (explained more fully in Chapter 7) must be especially careful to get enough omega-3s since their blood levels of this important nutrient tend to be only about half that of other pregnant women.

Omega-3 fatty acid, also called linolenic acid, can be found in

- all fish and seafood
- egg yolks
- the leaves and seeds of many plants
- soybeans
- nuts
- oils such as canola, flaxseed, olive, and walnut

Omega-6 fatty acids, also called linoleic acid, can be found in:

- nuts, including walnuts, peanuts, and almonds
- seeds such as sunflower seeds
- oils such as corn, safflower, sunflower, and soybean

Most people don't get enough of the essential fatty acids in their diets. Those who do tend to consume the less beneficial omega-6s (from the oils used in processed foods) rather than the more advantageous omega-3s. I suggest that you limit your intake of omega-6s, and aim for 1,000 milligrams of omega-3s every day.

Fish and seafood—salmon, albacore tuna, lake trout, anchovies, sardines, shrimp—are your best sources for omega-3s. In making your selection, remember that the fattier the fish, the higher the omega-3 fatty acid content. For example, a three-and-a-half-ounce serving of salmon has twice as much omega-3s as tuna, and six times as much as crab.

Do, however, check with your local health authority to make sure the fish sold in your area is free from contaminants. Follow their advice in selecting fresh, unpolluted fish. Limit your consumption of swordfish or shark to three times a month, because these larger fish tend to absorb more concentrated levels of toxic metals than smaller fish do. Also avoid raw fish, such as sushi. Always bake, broil, or steam your fish rather than frying, because the higher frying temperatures destroy the oils.

The right oils are also good sources of the essential fatty acids your baby needs. Best choices include olive, flaxseed, canola, and safflower oil. Use these in cooking and in salad dressings. Limit hydrogenated shortenings and butter.

Also try the new eggs that are enriched with vitamin E and omega-3 fatty acids, marketed under brand names such as Eggland's Best, Wilcox Farms, Golden-Premium, and the Golden Hen. These eggs come from chickens whose feed is fortified with vitamin E, flaxseed, and fish oils. Compared to regular eggs, these enriched eggs contain two to six times the amount of omega-3 fatty acids and vitamin E.

How Much Fat Do You Need?
About 30 to 40 percent of your daily calories should come from the good fats. This may surprise you, because the common advice is to limit fats to less than 30 percent of daily calories. During pregnancy, however, some women find that they cannot eat enough food at any one time to get all the calories they need. In these cases, a diet that includes up to 40 percent fat can supply a more concentrated source of nutrients and calories. If you're underweight, aim for the high end of the range shown below; if you're overweight, stick to the low end of the range:

- Get 67 to 89 grams of fat per day before you get pregnant.
- Get 73 to 98 grams of fat per day during the first trimester.
- Get 83 to 111 grams of fat per day during the second and third trimesters.
- Get 90 to 120 grams of fat per day during breastfeeding.

Table 2-5 provides a concise review of the requirements for all the macronutrients and calories needed before, during, and after pregnancy.

TABLE 2-5. CALORIC AND MACRONUTRIENT REQUIREMENTS BEFORE, DURING, AND AFTER PREGNANCY

Nutrients	Percent of Calories	Nonpregnant	Pregnant		Breastfeeding
			1ST TRIMESTER	2ND & 3RD TRIMESTERS	
Total calories (per day)		2,000	2,200	2,500	2,700
Protein (grams)	20–25%	100–125	110–138	125–156	135–169
Carbohydrate (grams)	40–50%	200–250	220–275	250–312	270–338
Fat (grams)	30–40%	67–89	73–98	83–111	90–120

WATER

During pregnancy, drinking water is one of the most important ways in which you can protect your baby, because *adequate hydration helps prevent premature labor.* Babies who are born prematurely are at increased risk for many problems, including hearing loss, vision loss, respiratory disorders, serious developmental disabilities, and even death.

Water helps both you and your baby. Here's how:

- Dehydration can trigger uterine contractions, which in turn can lead to premature birth. "Anytime I slacked off on my water intake, I got dehydrated and started having contractions," says Ally, a mother of twins. "But the contractions would stop once I sat down and drank a big glass of water."
- The hormonal changes that occur during pregnancy make you more prone to urinary tract infections, which can also trigger premature labor. Drinking plenty of water guards against this potential complication.
- During pregnancy your metabolism revs up. In the first trimester, before your blood volume increases, an adequate intake of fluids helps dissipate some of this additional body heat.
- Pregnancy hormones can leave you constipated. Drinking water improves regularity.
- Staying hydrated reduces your susceptibility to headaches, dry skin, and complexion problems.

Aim for *at least eight 16-ounce glasses of water—that's four quarts—every day*. Although taking in this much water every day may seem tough, it can be integrated into your daily routine as easily as any other healthy habit. One strategy is to keep water within easy reach at all times. Jean, a mother of three, says, "At the office I kept a bottle of water on my desk constantly, and I had a six-pack of water in my car. At home, my water bottles were everywhere—in the kitchen and the bathroom, on my night table, even in the laundry room. My husband teased me about tripping over them wherever he turned."

If you're not yet in the water habit, experiment and you'll soon figure out which way water tastes best to you. Some women prefer it icy cold; others like it at room temperature. Try a bit of flavor, too, by adding a lemon slice or splash of fruit juice to each glass.

Understand that this prescription for fluids means mostly H_2O. Fruit juices can cause wide swings in your blood sugar levels. Soft drinks, club soda, and other carbonated beverages may make your stomach uncomfortably bloated, leaving little room for the foods you and your baby need. Coffee and tea both contain caffeine, which acts as a diuretic and thereby contributes to dehydration. So stick to water. You'll soon develop a taste for it, if you haven't already. And there's a bonus: Keeping up this habit after you deliver will help you get your figure back more quickly.

The ABCs of Vitamins and Minerals

Vitamins and minerals are essential nutrients that aid various metabolic processes and help maintain the body's structural health. Vitamins and minerals do not contribute calories. Instead, they play vital roles in processing carbohydrates into energy, turning proteins into tissue for growth or healing, and converting fats into storage for energy use at a later time.

Vitamins and minerals are always needed in small amounts. During pregnancy, the daily requirements for nearly all vitamins and minerals increase. The Food and Nutrition Board of the National Institute of Medicine publishes Recommended Dietary Allowances (RDAs) for levels of intake that have been determined to be healthy. The most recent edition was issued in 1989. More recently, the Food and Nutrition Board has adopted a new approach, termed Dietary Reference Intakes (DRIs). These are designed to include the most current understanding of the role of nutrients and food components in long-term health.

VITAL VITAMINS FOR YOUR BABY

Your baby's metabolic programming is greatly affected by the supply of vitamins he or she receives through the foods you eat. Taken in the right amounts at the right times, vitamins help to protect your child from neural tube defects such as spina bifida, as well as from premature birth and low birthweight. They protect you, too, from high blood pressure and various other pregnancy complications.

The body needs vitamins for metabolism (the process of converting food to energy), for growth and development, and for the maintenance of good health. The thirteen essential vitamins that your body needs are divided into two groups: the fat-soluble vitamins and the water-soluble vitamins.

The fat-soluble vitamins, which are stored mainly in fatty tissues and the liver, include vitamins A, D, E, and K. The water-soluble vitamins, which are not stored in the body for very long, include vitamin C and the B vitamins: thiamin (vitamin B_1), riboflavin (vitamin B_2), niacin (vitamin B_3), pantothenic acid (vitamin B_5), pyridoxine (vitamin B_6), biotin (vitamin B_7), folic acid (vitamin B_9), and cobalamin (vitamin B_{12}).

Table 2-6 lists the RDA or DRI for each vitamin, with separate recommendations for pregnant women (the first number) and for nursing mothers (the second number). The table also includes a list of good dietary sources for each vitamin.

The menus I've provided in this book are designed to allow you to meet all the RDAs. If you decide to create your own menus, please make sure that your daily diet provides appropriate amounts of each of these thirteen important vitamins.

Understand, too, that when it comes to vitamins, more is not necessarily better. In fact, *when consumed in doses that are too high, vitamins can interfere with the metabolism of other nutrients and even cause birth defects.* For example:

TABLE 2-6. GOOD DIETARY SOURCES OF VITAMINS

Nutrient	Daily Value	RDA or DRI	GOOD FOOD SOURCES						
			Fruits	Vegetables	Cereals and Nuts	Meats	Fish	Poultry	Dairy
Vitamin A	4,000 IU	4,000 IU 6,500 IU	Cantaloupe Mangoes Peaches	Carrots Squash Greens Pumpkin Sweet potatoes Spinach		Liver	Salmon Tuna		Cheese Eggs Milk
Vitamin B$_1$ (Thiamin)	1.5 mg	1.4 mg 1.4 mg	Oranges	Peas Beans	Wheat germ Pastas Oatmeal Cereals Breads	Pork Beef			
Vitamin B$_2$ (Riboflavin)	1.7 mg	1.4 mg 1.6 mg		Asparagus Broccoli Collard greens Spinach Turnip greens	Cereals	Beef liver	Fish	Chicken Turkey	Cheese Milk Yogurt
Vitamin B$_3$ (Niacin)	20 mg	18 mg 17 mg		Potatoes	Cereals Peanut butter	Beef Veal	Salmon Tuna	Chicken	

Vitamin									
Vitamin B₅ (Pantothenic acid)		6 mg 7 mg		Beans	Whole grains	Beef Liver Pork	Fish	Chicken	
Vitamin B₆ (Pyridoxine)	2 mg	1.9 mg 2.0 mg	Avocados Bananas		Brown rice Soybeans Oats Whole wheat Peanuts Walnuts	Beef	Fish	Chicken	Eggs
Vitamin B₇ (Biotin)		30 µg 35 µg	Bananas		Oatmeal Peanut butter	Liver	Clams Salmon		Eggs
Vitamin B₉ (Folic acid)	400 mcg	600 mcg 500 mcg	Oranges	Asparagus Beans Beets Broccoli Spinach Romaine lettuce	Cereals	Beef liver			
Vitamin B₁₂ (Cobalamin)	6 mcg	2.6 mcg 2.8 mcg				Beef liver Pork	Clams Crab Herring Oysters Salmon Tuna		Milk Yogurt

GOOD FOOD SOURCES

Nutrient	Daily Value	RDA or DRI	Fruits	Vegetables	Cereals and Nuts	Meats	Fish	Poultry	Dairy
Vitamin C	60 mg	85 mg 120 mg	Cantaloupe Pineapple Oranges Strawberries Grapefruit	Broccoli Collard greens Peppers					
Vitamin D	400 IU	400 IU 400 IU			Cereals		Herring Mackerel Shrimp Sardines Salmon		Milk Eggs
Vitamin E		15 mg 19 mg		Corn oil Soybean oil Safflower oil Spinach	Whole grains Wheat germ				
Vitamin K	65 µg	65 µg 65 µg		Cauliflower Broccoli Spinach Cabbage		Beef liver			

- The RDA for vitamin A is 4,000 IU. Daily doses of 10,000 IU can cause congenital malformations. Doses of 25,000 IU can lead to miscarriage early in pregnancy.
- The RDA for vitamin D is 400 IU. Daily doses of 4,000 IU can result in birth defects.
- Large doses of vitamin C interfere with the body's ability to use vitamin B_{12}.
- Large doses of vitamin B_6 impede the body's ability to use vitamin B_2.
- Vitamins D and E, in excess, interfere with vitamin A.

The Power of Folic Acid

One particular vitamin is so powerful in preventing pregnancy problems that we need to discuss it at greater length. This vitamin is folic acid, also called vitamin B_9.

Each year in the United States about four thousand pregnancies are affected by serious birth defects of the spine and brain, known as neural tube defects. Not long ago, it was discovered that folic acid reduces this risk by 50 percent or more. *However, folic acid can protect against neural tube defects only in the very early stages of pregnancy.* To promote your baby's positive programming, you must ensure that your intake of folic acid is adequate even before you conceive or, if that's not possible, as soon as you realize you're pregnant.

Folic acid may protect your baby from other threats as well. Some studies show a connection between low blood levels of this vitamin and an increased risk for Down's syndrome (a combination of mental retardation and physical abnormalities caused by the presence of an extra chromosome)[3,4]. Other studies reveal that folic acid deficiency is associated with a twofold risk of premature birth and of birthweights of less than 5.5 pounds[5].

The power of this vitamin to protect unborn babies is so indisputable that in 1992 the Centers for Disease Control issued a national recommendation: All women of childbearing age who are capable of becoming pregnant should consume folic acid every day[6]. The daily requirement is:

- 400 micrograms a day for all women of childbearing age
- 600 micrograms a day for pregnant women
- 500 micrograms a day for women who are breastfeeding

Unfortunately, many women have not received this message. According to a Gallup poll commissioned by the March of Dimes Birth Defects Foundation in 1998, only 13 percent of women ages 18 to 45 knew that folic acid prevents birth defects, and only 7 percent knew that folic acid should be taken before you become pregnant, as well as during your pregnancy. It's also important to know that deficiencies of vitamin B_{12} and the mineral zinc can impair your body's ability to use folic acid. Your intake of these two nutrients, therefore, also must be adequate.

The richest natural sources of folic acid are oranges and orange juice, asparagus, beets, broccoli, spinach, and romaine lettuce. However, the natural form of this vitamin is not as well absorbed as the synthetic form. That's one reason why the U.S. Food and Drug Administration (FDA) mandated in 1998 that folic acid be added to grain-based staples such as bread, pasta, and rice, and also authorized ready-to-eat cereals to be fully fortified up to 100 percent of the RDA per serving. This level of fortification has already led to improved blood levels of this important nutrient in the American population[7]. Supplements in pill form are also widely available. But again, more is not always better—the safe upper limit for folic acid is 1,000 micrograms daily.

Multivitamin Supplements

When you're pregnant, think of a multivitamin supplement as a nutritional insurance policy for your baby's positive metabolic programming. Studies show that *the risk for birth defects of the cardiovascular system and urinary tract, as well as for cleft lip and cleft palate, can be dramatically reduced with the daily intake of a multivitamin containing folic acid* during the period from one month before through two months after conception[8,9,10,11,12,13,14].

I advise that you take a multivitamin supplement that contains *only vitamins* (not minerals), and at the level of no more than 100 to 150 percent of the RDA. Many such preparations are available; my favorite is One A Day Essentials. If swallowing pills is a problem for you, try children's chewable multivitamins. Usually, two children's tablets will equal an adult's daily requirement, but check the label to be sure.

In recommending a multivitamin, I am in no way suggesting that it's all right to get lax about your food choices. Your diet is your primary armamentarium for getting all the nutrients you need each day. But I realize that some days it's hard to eat exactly as you should. In certain circumstances you need to be especially conscientious about taking a multivitamin. You should take a multivitamin if:

- you don't eat the recommended number of fruits and vegetables on a regular basis
- you're under a lot of stress at work or at home, particularly for long periods
- you're recovering from surgery or a prolonged or serious illness
- you have a chronic condition such as asthma or diabetes
- you've been taking medication over a long period of time
- you smoked before you got pregnant
- you drank alcohol on a regular basis before getting pregnant

What about the prenatal vitamin-mineral supplements that obstetricians sometimes prescribe? I am not in favor of taking these because, when vitamins and minerals are combined in one tablet, the body's ability to absorb them is limited. Also, these tablets typically contain vitamins and minerals at levels two to four times the RDA, which is unnecessary and perhaps risky. These

supplements can add to the nausea and vomiting of early pregnancy, and they may decrease your appetite, leaving you less
able to eat the foods your unborn baby needs. Prenatal vitamin-
mineral supplements also can cause irregularity. Jean, one of my
patients, says, "The prenatal tablets my doctor gave me made me
so constipated that I was in misery. When I switched to a vitamin-
only supplement, I felt a lot better."

ALL ABOUT MINERALS
Minerals contribute significantly to your baby's positive programming, and also to the degree of good health you will enjoy during
your pregnancy. For instance, adequate intake of the appropriate
minerals can:

- aid in the proper development of your baby's nervous system
- reduce the risk of preterm labor
- guard against infection
- help prevent hypertension during pregnancy

We need certain minerals in amounts over 100 mg per day, while
for others (called trace minerals) the requirements are lower—yet
both types are equally important to good health. The minerals we
need every day include calcium, magnesium, phosphorus, and
potassium. The important trace minerals include chromium, cop-
per, iodine, iron, manganese, selenium, and zinc. In Table 2-7
you'll find the RDA or DRI for each mineral, with separate recommendations for pregnant women (the first number) and for nursing mothers (the second number). This table also includes a list of
good dietary sources for each mineral.

Iron: Are You Deficient?
Your red blood cells carry oxygen to all the tissues of your body—
and to your unborn baby. If your blood level of iron is too low, the
oxygen-carrying capacity of the red blood cells is compromised,

and your baby cannot receive the oxygen he or she needs for optimal growth and development.

Unfortunately, iron deficiency is very common. In fact, it's the single most prevalent nutritional deficiency in the world. It is most often found among individuals who are at peak rates of growth: infants, young children, and pregnant women. According to the World Health Organization, the problem is worst in developing countries, with 35 to 75 percent of women lacking sufficient iron, but it also occurs among 20 percent of women in developed countries.

Many women are already iron deficient before they conceive and then become severely anemic due to the high iron demands of pregnancy. This can cause a significant slowing of fetal growth, particularly when it occurs in the first trimester[15]. Iron deficiency also can make you feel fatigued, light-headed, and short of breath.

I tell my patients that an iron-rich diet is the best safeguard against such problems. The top sources of iron are beef, pork, chicken, lamb, fish, and eggs. The type of iron these foods contain is known as *heme iron*, which is well absorbed by the body and is not affected by other factors in your diet.

Certain plant foods such as spinach, beans, potatoes, and enriched grains and cereals contain a type of iron called *non-heme iron*. This is poorly absorbed, particularly when eaten along with foods containing calcium and fiber. Absorption of non-heme iron can be improved by combining it with foods rich in vitamin C or animal protein.

When you're pregnant, you can be sure your diet contains adequate iron if you are eating 6 ounces of meat, fish, or poultry plus one fresh egg, or seven servings of meat equivalents each day.

There is currently some controversy in the United States regarding iron supplementation during pregnancy. The World Health Organization and the Institute of Medicine recommend supplements, while the U.S. Preventive Medicine Task Force does not. I do not recommend that you take iron supplements while you're

TABLE 2-7. GOOD DIETARY SOURCES OF MINERALS

GOOD FOOD SOURCES

Nutrient	Daily Value	RDA or DRI	Fruits	Vegetables	Cereals and Nuts	Meats	Fish	Poultry	Dairy
Calcium	1,000 mg	1,000 mg 1,000 mg	Calcium-fortified orange juice	Broccoli Collard greens Kale Mustard greens Tofu	Corn tortillas processed with lime		Salmon Sardines		Milk Cheese Yogurt
Chromium	120 mcg		Apples Grapes	Corn Broccoli Sweet potatoes		Beef Pork			Eggs
Copper	2 mg		Avocados	Beans Mushrooms Potatoes	Nuts Seeds Whole grains	Beef liver	Shellfish		
Iodine	150 mcg				Breads		Lobster Shrimp Oysters		Milk
Iron	18 mg	30 mg 15 mg	Raisins	Beans Spinach Potatoes	Wheat cereal	Beef Lamb Pork	Clams		
Magnesium	400 mcg	350 mcg 310 mcg	Avocados Bananas	Beans Broccoli	Peanuts Brown rice		Haddock		Milk Yogurt

Mineral	Amount	Fruits	Vegetables	Grains / Nuts	Meat	Shellfish	Poultry	Dairy
Manganese	2 mg	Pineapple	Collard greens, Potatoes, Spinach	Oatmeal				
Phosphorus	700 mg, 700 mg		Carrots, Broccoli, Spinach	Wheat bran, Wheat germ, Whole grains, Nuts, Seeds	Beef liver	Shellfish	Chicken	Milk, Eggs, Yogurt
Potassium	3,500 mg	Avocados, Apricots, Prunes, Bananas, Cantaloupe	Potatoes, Spinach, Beans					Milk
Selenium	70 mcg, 60 mg, 70 mg			Whole grains, Brazil nuts	Beef, Liver	Clams, Crab, Oysters, Lobster		
Zinc	12 mg, 15 mg, 19 mg		Beans	Whole grains, Nuts	Beef, Lamb	Oysters	Turkey	Eggs, Yogurt

pregnant. My primary reason is that iron pills can cause constipation and exacerbate nausea and vomiting, and these conditions can prevent you from eating (or keeping down) the foods your unborn baby needs. It also takes more than iron to build your blood.

If your healthcare provider does recommend an iron supplement, you should take it on an empty stomach or with a snack that does not include dairy products, so that it's more readily absorbed. *Do not take iron and calcium supplements at the same time of day.* A good rule of thumb is to take your calcium supplement at least one hour before or two hours after you take the iron supplement.

◀ *If you're planning to get pregnant,* you should know that iron deficiency may be associated with infertility[16]. Also, if you're anemic now, you have a higher risk of becoming severely anemic during pregnancy. To prevent these problems, eat an iron-rich diet. If you need help in planning iron-rich meals, ask your doctor for a referral to a registered dietitian.

Calcium, Magnesium, and Zinc

The majority of adult women in the United States do not meet the RDAs for calcium, magnesium, or zinc, according to the USDA[17]. Yet these three minerals are essential for your baby.

- Calcium significantly reduces your risk of developing preeclampsia, a dangerous complication of pregnancy that is more common among women pregnant for the first time, as well as those who are expecting twins or supertwins.
- Magnesium helps to prevent premature labor by minimizing uterine contractions. It also lowers your baby's risk of cerebral palsy or mental retardation after birth, because it protects the developing nervous system.
- Zinc is vital for the healthy development of your baby's ner-

vous system. Plus, it reduces the occurrence of infection during pregnancy.
- These minerals also make you more comfortable by reducing heartburn, leg cramps, and insomnia.

TABLE 2-8. PER CAPITA CONSUMPTION OF MAJOR FOODS*

(In pounds)	1970	1975	1980	1985	1990	1995
Red meat	131.7	125.8	126.4	124.9	112.3	114.7
Fish and shellfish	11.7	12.1	12.4	15.0	15.0	14.9
Poultry	33.8	32.9	40.8	45.5	56.3	62.9
Yogurt	0.8	2.1	2.6	4.1	4.1	5.1
Cheese	11.4	14.3	17.5	22.5	24.6	27.3
Butter	5.4	4.7	4.5	4.9	4.4	4.5
Margarine	10.8	11.0	11.3	10.8	10.9	9.1
(In gallons)	**1970**	**1975**	**1980**	**1985**	**1990**	**1995**
Whole milk	21.7	21.0	17.0	14.3	10.5	8.8
Lowfat/skim milk	5.3	8.3	10.5	12.3	15.2	15.6
Bottled water	—	—	2.4	4.5	8.0	11.6
Diet soft drinks	2.1	3.2	5.1	7.1	10.7	11.8
Regular soft drinks	22.2	25.0	29.9	28.7	35.6	39.8
Beer	30.6	33.9	36.6	34.6	34.4	31.6
Wine	2.2	2.7	3.2	3.5	2.9	2.6
Distilled spirits	3.0	3.1	3.0	2.6	2.2	1.8

*Adapted from USDA

I'm not surprised that calcium is among the minerals women are most likely to lack, because few adults drink adequate amounts of milk. In fact, as you can see in Table 2-8, people in the United States drink twice as much soda as milk, and 50 percent more beer, wine, and spirits than milk. Yet contrary to what some people believe, milk is an excellent choice for adults. If you avoid milk because you are lactose intolerant, as many adults are, buy lactose-free milk instead of regular milk.

Your goal during pregnancy is to get 2 grams of calcium per day. You can achieve this by getting the recommended four to six servings of dairy foods daily. Also, boost your intake of calcium-rich foods such as yogurt, cheese, salmon, broccoli, and tofu. Calcium-fortified orange juice is another good option.

You also need to make sure you're getting at least 800 mg of magnesium per day. Your four to six servings of dairy foods will help. In addition, you should eat eight servings of fruits and vegetables (good choices include bananas, beans, spinach, and avocados) as well as eight servings of grains (rich sources are oatmeal and brown rice).

For zinc, your goal is 30 mg per day. You can reach that level by eating the recommended six servings of protein foods (beef, lamb, turkey, eggs), your four servings of dairy foods, and your eight servings of grains.

Because deficiencies of these three minerals are so common and yet so risky during pregnancy, I also recommend that you take a multimineral supplement that contains calcium, magnesium, and zinc. These are available from a number of manufacturers. Look for brands that contain 333 mg of calcium carbonate, 133 mg magnesium oxide, and 5 mg zinc oxide per tablet. You should take two tablets three times a day: after lunch, after dinner, and after your bedtime snack. These last two doses correspond with the times of day when uterine contractions are most likely to occur, so the increase of these minerals in your blood levels will help to counteract that risk.

For my patients pregnant with twins, triplets, or quadruplets, I increase the dosage to 3 grams of calcium, 1.2 grams of magnesium, and 45 mg of zinc daily—that's nine tablets total per day—

for the babies' sake as well as the mother's. "The calcium, magnesium, and zinc supplements really eased my nausea and indigestion," says Rebecca, a mother of twin boys. "They were also wonderful for leg cramps. In fact, I soon realized that I only got the cramps when I'd forgotten to take the supplements."

If you choose to include only a calcium supplement, select calcium carbonate or calcium citrate for best absorption. Calcium carbonate is the most concentrated and economical form of calcium. And remember, calcium is most easily absorbed when taken with food. Many women rely on an over-the-counter heartburn remedy such as Tums to provide calcium, but I don't recommend this practice. Too much calcium carbonate can cause "rebound hyperacidity," or excess stomach acid. Also avoid calcium supplements made from oyster shells or dolomite; these may be contaminated with lead or other heavy metals.

ANTIOXIDANTS: A RECENT DISCOVERY

Besides vitamins and minerals, there are other substances that can help prevent disease and promote health—the bioflavinoids, which were discovered only in the last few decades. Part of the larger family of plant phytochemicals, they are potent antioxidants that also give fruits and vegetables their bright colors. They include:

- thioesters (garlic, onions, leeks)
- terpenes (citrus fruits)
- plant phenols (grapes, strawberries, apples)
- carotenoids (carrots, yams, sweet potatoes, watermelon)
- lutein (tomatoes)

The most nutritious fruits and vegetables are those that are fresh; frozen and canned varieties are fine, too. Don't fool yourself: Ketchup does not count as a vegetable serving, because processing robs foods of their nutrients. As long as you're eating the recommended amounts of fruits and vegetables, you're getting the bioflavinoids you and your baby need.

◄ *If you're planning to get pregnant,* now is the perfect time to improve your diet, focusing on the specific nutrients in which you may be deficient. That's because the first weeks immediately following conception are a critical time in an unborn baby's metabolic programming. Dietary changes made now boost the odds that your baby will have an optimal nutrition environment, right from the very moment of conception.

Your Prepregnancy Weight: Why It Matters Now

A healthy weight is more than just a number on the bathroom scale. It's a balance between your body's proportions of muscle and fat. When you're trying to get pregnant, your weight can influence this whether or not you conceive. The amount of body fat associated with regular menstrual periods and overall good health ranges from 20 to 30 percent, with proportions outside this range being associated with fertility and pregnancy problems[18,19,20]. Once you are pregnant, your weight directly affects how healthy your baby will be at birth.

Body fat is difficult to measure, so clinicians use several simple procedures to estimate it. The oldest method is weight-for-height, used by many life insurance companies to define mortality risks (see Table 2-9). Based on a comparison to normal weight-for-height and frame size, underweight is considered to be 10 percent or more below normal, while overweight is 20 percent or more above normal.

TABLE 2-9. PREPREGNANCY WEIGHT-FOR-HEIGHT AND BODY FRAME SIZE

Height (inches)	SMALL FRAME			MEDIUM FRAME			LARGE FRAME		
	Underweight	Normal Weight	Overweight	Underweight	Normal Weight	Overweight	Underweight	Normal Weight	Overweight
57	94	104	125	100	112	134	109	122	146
58	95	105	126	102	114	137	112	124	149
59	96	107	128	105	117	140	114	127	152
60	98	109	131	107	119	143	116	129	155
61	101	112	134	110	122	146	118	132	158
62	104	115	138	113	125	150	122	136	163
63	106	118	142	115	128	154	126	140	168
64	109	121	145	118	131	157	128	143	172
65	112	124	149	120	134	161	132	147	176
66	114	127	152	123	137	164	135	150	180
67	117	130	156	126	140	168	138	154	185
68	120	133	160	129	143	172	141	157	188
69	122	136	163	131	146	175	144	160	192
70	125	139	167	134	149	179	146	163	196
71	128	142	170	137	152	182	149	166	199
72	131	145	174	140	155	186	152	169	203

A second method for gauging body fat is the body mass index, or BMI, which more accurately describes the relationship between height and weight (see Table 2-10). To calculate your prepregnancy body mass index, locate your height in the far left column, then move across that row to find your weight. At the top of your weight column is your body mass index. A BMI in the range of 20 to 25 is considered healthy; below 20 is underweight; above 25 is overweight; and above 29 is obese.

The third measure is waist-to-hip ratio, or WHR. This measure identifies the proportion of upper-body fat to lower-body fat. To determine your waist-to-hip ratio, divide your waist measurement by your hip measurement. A waist-to-hip ratio greater than 0.8 is considered a health risk, particularly for heart disease.

Your recommended weight gain during pregnancy is discussed in detail in Chapter 6. But here's a preview of what you should aim for:

- If you were of normal weight before becoming pregnant, your total weight gain should be 25 to 35 pounds.
- If you began this pregnancy already overweight, your total weight gain should be about 15 to 25 pounds.
- If you were underweight when you conceived, aim to gain a total of 28 to 40 pounds.

◀ *If you're planning to get pregnant,* and you're overweight, you should try to *lose enough weight to get within the ideal range before you conceive—but don't go on a crash diet* that restricts you to less than 1,200 calories per day, or any diet that relies on special foods or dietary supplements. These put you at risk for depleting your body's reserves of vital nutrients, particularly iron, thereby doing you (and your baby-to-be) more harm than good.

TABLE 2-10. DETERMINING YOUR BODY MASS INDEX (BMI)

BODY MASS INDEX

BODY WEIGHT (LB)

Height (inches)	17	18	19	20	21	22	23	24	25	26	27	28	29	30	31	32	33	34	35
58	82	87	91	96	100	105	110	115	119	124	129	134	138	143	149	154	159	163	168
59	85	90	94	99	104	109	114	119	124	128	133	138	143	148	154	159	164	169	174
60	87	93	97	102	107	112	118	123	128	133	138	143	148	153	159	165	170	175	180
61	90	96	100	106	111	116	122	127	132	137	143	148	153	158	165	170	175	181	186
62	93	99	104	109	115	120	126	131	136	142	147	153	158	164	170	176	181	187	192
63	96	102	107	113	118	124	130	135	141	146	152	158	163	169	176	181	187	193	198
64	99	105	110	116	122	128	134	140	145	151	157	163	169	174	181	187	193	199	205
65	103	109	114	120	126	132	138	144	150	156	162	168	174	180	187	193	199	205	211
66	106	112	118	124	130	136	142	148	155	161	167	173	179	186	193	199	205	212	218
67	109	115	121	127	134	140	146	153	159	166	172	178	185	191	199	205	211	218	224
68	112	119	125	131	138	144	151	158	164	171	177	184	190	197	205	211	218	225	231
69	116	122	128	135	142	149	155	162	169	176	182	189	196	203	211	218	224	231	238
70	119	126	132	139	146	153	160	167	174	181	188	195	202	207	217	224	230	238	245
71	122	130	136	143	150	157	165	172	179	186	193	200	208	215	223	230	238	244	252
72	126	133	140	147	154	162	169	177	184	191	199	206	213	221	230	237	244	251	259
73	129	137	144	151	159	166	174	182	189	197	204	212	219	227	236	244	251	259	266
74	133	141	148	155	163	171	179	186	194	202	210	218	225	233	243	250	258	266	274
	UNDERWEIGHT			NORMAL WEIGHT						OVERWEIGHT				OBESE					

There are 3,500 calories in a pound of body fat, so by reducing your daily intake by 500 calories, you can lose one pound per week. This is a good rate at which to lose weight while still maintaining your energy levels and nutrient stores. Many reducing diets are currently available. The safest are those based on the daily consumption of a variety of healthful foods, as well as ample fluid and adequate fiber. My favorite reducing diets include the Zone and Weight Watchers. Also, refer to the Reducing Diet Plan at the end of this chapter, in the section called Menus for Before You Get Pregnant. This plan provides a week's worth of sample menus that provide a daily intake of 1,200 calories.

◄ *If you're planning to get pregnant,* and *you're underweight,* you can achieve a healthy rate of weight gain—about 1 to 1½ pounds per week—by eating an additional 500 to 750 calories daily. These additional calories should come from foods that help build up your nutrient stores. Avoid selections that provide little more than empty calories, such as chocolate, candy, soda, and chips.

Instead, go for foods rich in vitamins, minerals, fiber, or protein, such as lean meats, fish, poultry, dairy products (yogurt, cheeses, milk, milkshakes, ice cream, and frozen yogurt), cereals and grains, and fruits and vegetables. Here are examples of foods that contribute 500 to 750 calories per day:

- 8 ounces of lowfat yogurt and a toasted waffle with one tablespoon peanut butter
- a quarter-pound hamburger with cheese
- two slices of French toast with two ounces of cheddar cheese
- a 12-ounce malted milkshake

Super-Powered Drinks: The Nutritional Supplements

Nutritional supplements are specially formulated foods, available in beverage and pudding form (not to be confused with vitamin and mineral supplements in tablet or capsule form discussed above). They are nutritionally balanced, calorically concentrated, and easy to digest, and can be found in pharmacies and grocery stores. Brand names include Ensure, Instant Breakfast, Sweet Success, Boost, Sustacal, ReSource, Deliver 2.0, and TwoCal HN. For certain pregnant women, these supplements provide an extra boost of high-powered nutrition to help both mother and baby to thrive.

I strongly recommend adding nutritional supplements to your daily diet in the following circumstances:

- if you think you are deficient in any of the important nutrients discussed above
- if you're underweight
- if you have lost weight due to severe morning sickness, food poisoning, or any other illness
- if your doctor is concerned that your pregnancy weight gain is insufficient
- if you're a smoker or an ex-smoker
- if you're pregnant with triplets or quadruplets
- if you are in your third trimester and feel full too quickly to eat a complete meal

The major advantage of nutritional supplements is that they are the most concentrated, nutritionally balanced, easily absorbed form of food. As such, they can be the key to turbo-boosting your nutritional status. Their major disadvantage is that they can fill you up and may decrease your appetite for other foods.

There are basically three types of supplements. To help you

understand their nutritional content, I've compared them to a glass of whole milk. First, there are the regular supplements, which, for the same serving size, provide one-third to two-thirds more calories than a glass of milk, plus 50 percent more protein and three times as much carbohydrate. Including two or three servings of these supplements per day will boost your caloric intake by about 400 to 750 calories.

In the next group are the high-calorie supplements and the high-protein supplements. These supply about twice the protein and calories as a glass of whole milk, and four times the carbohydrate. Two or three servings per day will add 500 to 1,000 calories to your daily diet. These first two types of nutritional supplements are your best choices because they come in a range of flavors (including vanilla, chocolate, strawberry, banana, eggnog, and butterscotch), which keeps them from becoming boring day after day. Also, they are widely available in supermarkets, so you can stock up on them when you do your weekly grocery shopping.

The last group of supplements I call the "big guns" because, ounce per ounce, they pack the biggest nutritional punch. These supplements are both high calorie and high protein, and are the most useful for improving your nutritional status as quickly as possible, and with the smallest quantity of food. Compared to whole milk, these supplements provide more than three times the calories, two to three times the protein and fat, and more than four times the carbohydrates. Two or three servings per day will add 900 to 1,400 calories to your diet, and as much as 60 grams of high-quality protein—the equivalent of 20 ounces of steak! Although the price is about the same as the high-calorie or high-protein supplements, they are not as readily available in local stores, and they only come in one flavor (vanilla). You can ask your pharmacist to order some for you to try.

A comparison of the three types of nutritional supplements is given in Table 2-11. All of these supplements are available directly from the manufacturers. If you order by phone using a credit

TABLE 2-11. COMPARISON OF NUTRITIONAL SUPPLEMENTS (PER SERVING)

	Calories	Protein (grams)	Carbohydrate (grams)	Fat (grams)	Flavors
WHOLE MILK (8 OZ.)	150	8	12	8	PLAIN
Regular Supplements					
Sweet Success	200	11	38	3	Vanilla, chocolate, strawberry, strawberry-banana
Instant Breakfast	200	12	31	3	Vanilla, chocolate
Boost	240	10	40	4	Vanilla, chocolate
Sustacal	240	14.5	33	5.5	Vanilla, chocolate, strawberry, eggnog
Ensure	250	8.8	40	6.1	Vanilla, chocolate
ReSource	250	9	34	9	Vanilla, chocolate, strawberry
ReSource Fruit Beverage	180	9	36	0	Fruit-flavored
High-Calorie or High-Protein Supplements					
Sustacal Pudding	240	6.8	32	9.5	Vanilla, chocolate, butterscotch
Ensure Pudding	250	6.8	34	9.7	Vanilla, chocolate, butterscotch, tapioca
Sustacal Plus	360	14.4	45	13.6	Vanilla, chocolate, strawberry, eggnog
Ensure Plus	355	13	47.3	12.6	Vanilla, chocolate, strawberry
Ensure Plus HN	355	14.8	47.3	11.8	Vanilla, chocolate
ReSource Plus	360	13	47	13	Vanilla, chocolate
High-Calorie and High-Protein Supplements					
Deliver 2.0	470	17.7	47	24	Vanilla
TwoCal HN	475	19.8	51.4	21.5	Vanilla

card, they will be delivered directly to your door and shipping is free. My advice is to buy several cans in your local store, see if you like the taste, then order them in quantity. It's best to include a supplement between meals and before bedtime, and even more frequently if possible. The cost of these nutritional supplements can add up, so ask your obstetrician to write you a prescription, or work with a nutritionist or registered dietitian to explore whether they might be covered by your health insurance.

◀ *If you're planning to get pregnant,* and you're underweight, you might want to start using nutritional supplements now to jumpstart your weight gain. This is particularly wise if you have trouble gaining weight, are recovering from illness, or are an ex-smoker.

Food Safety: A Word of Caution

If you've ever had food poisoning, or thought you had food poisoning, you know what it's like to feel deathly ill for hours or even days. Certainly it's something you need to avoid at all times, but particularly when you're pregnant. The key is to be careful of what you choose to eat, and in how you handle food.

A summary of the major types of food poisoning, including causes and symptoms, can be found in Table 2-12. For more information, contact the Food Safety and Inspection Service Meat and Poultry Hotline at 1-800-535-4555, the USDA Food Information Hotline at 1-888-SAFEFOOD, or log on to the Food Safety and Inspection Service Web site at http://www.fsis.usda.gov.

FOOD HANDLING AND PREPARATION TIPS

Bacteria grow slowly at low temperatures, multiply rapidly at midrange temperatures, and are killed at high temperatures. For food to be safe, it must be cooked to an internal temperature high enough to destroy harmful bacteria. According to the USDA, temperature is the only way to gauge whether food is sufficiently cooked. Appearance and "touch tests" are not accurate. That's why a good meat thermometer is an indispensable kitchen item. The meat thermometer should be placed in the thickest part of the meat, away from bone, fat, or gristle.

Second, every kitchen needs at least two cutting boards, one reserved just for raw meats, fish, and poultry, and another for fresh fruits and vegetables. Cutting boards can harbor bacteria in cracks and grooves caused by knives, so choose ones that are smooth, durable, and can be cleaned easily. Wash them in hot soapy water, using a scrub brush to remove food particles. Afterward, sanitize acrylic boards by placing them in the dishwasher; rinse wooden boards with a dilute solution of one tablespoon bleach mixed with one gallon of water.

Wash your hands with warm soapy water before and after touching raw meat. Thoroughly cleanse any utensils that come in contact with raw meat, and never put cooked meat back onto a platter that held raw meat. Thoroughly reheat all meats purchased at deli counters before eating them. Keep your countertops and refrigerator clean, and be sure to observe the "use by" dates on food labels.

Poultry and Stuffing

As soon as you buy chicken or turkey, take it home and either refrigerate or freeze it. Cook the refrigerated bird within two days. Frozen poultry can be safely stored in your freezer for three months. Defrost poultry in the refrigerator, allowing twenty-four hours per five pounds. To thaw more quickly, put the bird in cold water, allowing thirty minutes per pound, and changing the water every thirty minutes. If you thaw poultry in the microwave, cook it immediately.

The safest way to prepare stuffing for poultry is to cook it separately. However, if you prefer to cook the stuffing in the bird, follow these guidelines. Prepare the stuffing just before it goes

TABLE 2-12. TYPES OF FOOD POISONING

Foodborne Pathogen	Sources	Mode of Transmission	Symptoms
Campylobacter jejuni	Intestinal tracts of animals and birds, raw milk, untreated water, and sewage sludge	Contaminated water, raw milk, and raw or undercooked meat, poultry, or shellfish	Fever, headache, and muscle pain followed by diarrhea (sometimes bloody), abdominal pain and nausea that appears 2 to 5 days after eating and lasting 7 to 10 days.
Clostridium botulinum	Widely distributed in nature; soil, water, on plants, and intestinal tracts of animals and fish. Grows only in little or no oxygen.	Bacteria produce a toxin that causes illness. Improperly canned foods, garlic in oil, vacuum-packed and tightly wrapped foods.	Toxin affects the nervous system. Symptoms usually appear 18 to 36 hours after consumption, but can sometimes appear as few as 4 hours or as many as 8 days after eating; double vision, droopy eyelids, trouble speaking and swallowing, and difficulty breathing. Fatal in 3 to 10 days if not treated.
Clostridium perfringens	Dust, soil, sewage, and intestinal tracts of animals and humans. Grows only in little or no oxygen.	Called the "cafeteria germ" because many outbreaks result from food left for long periods in steam tables or at room temperature. Bacteria is destroyed by cooking, but some toxin-producing spores may survive.	Diarrhea and gas pains may appear 8 to 24 hours after eating, usually lasting about 1 day, but less severe symptoms may persist for 1 to 2 weeks.

Organism	Source	Symptoms
Escherichia coli (E. coli)	Intestinal tracts of some mammals, raw milk, unchlorinated water	Contaminated water, raw milk, raw or rare ground beef, unpasteurized apple juice or cider, uncooked fruits and vegetables; person-to-person	Diarrhea or bloody diarrhea, abdominal cramps, nausea, malaise; can begin 2 to 5 days after food is eaten, lasting about 8 days. Some, especially the very young, have developed Hemolytic Uremic Syndrome that causes acute kidney failure. A similar illness, thrombocytopenic purpura, may occur in older adults.
Listeria monocytogenes	Intestinal tracts of humans and animals, milk, soil, leafy vegetables, and processed foods; can grow slowly at refrigerator temperatures	Soft cheese, raw milk, improperly processed ice cream, raw leafy vegetables, meat, and poultry. Illness is caused by bacteria that do not produce toxin.	Fever, chills, headache, backache, sometimes abdominal pain and diarrhea within 12 hours to 3 weeks. May later develop more serious illness in at-risk patients (meningitis or spontaneous abortion in pregnant women); sometimes just fatigue.
Salmonella	Intestinal tract and feces of animals; *Salmonella enteritidis* in raw eggs	Raw or undercooked eggs, poultry, and meat; raw milk and dairy products; seafood and food handlers	Stomach pain, diarrhea, nausea, chills, fever, and headache usually appear 8 to 72 hours after eating; may last 1 to 2 days.

Foodborne Pathogen	Sources	Mode of Transmission	Symptoms
Shigella	Human intestinal tract; rarely found in other animals	Person-to-person transmission by the fecal-oral route; fecal contamination of food and water. Most outbreaks result from food, especially salads, prepared and handled by workers using poor personal hygiene.	Disease referred to as "shigellosis" or bacillary dysentary. Diarrhea containing blood and mucus, fever, abdominal cramps, chills, vomiting; 12 to 50 hours from ingestion of bacteria; can last a few days to 2 weeks.
Staphylococcus aureus	On humans (skin, infected cuts, pimples, noses, and throats)	People to food through improper food handling. Multiply rapidly at room temperature to produce a toxin that causes illness.	Severe nausea, abdominal cramps, vomiting, and diarrhea occur within 1 to 6 hours after eating; recovery within 2 to 3 days, or longer if severe dehydration occurs.

into the bird. Make sure the stuffing is moist, because moist heat destroys bacteria more rapidly than dry heat. Pack stuffing loosely, about ¾ cup of stuffing per pound of meat. Immediately after you stuff the bird, place it in a preheated 325° F. oven. To gauge doneness, use a regular meat thermometer to ensure that the stuffing itself reaches an internal temperature of 165° F. and the poultry meat reaches 180° F. in the innermost part of the thigh. Don't rely on a pop-up thermometer, which does not measure the temperature of the stuffing inside the bird. The juices should run clear. Let the cooked bird stand outside the oven for twenty minutes before you remove the stuffing and carve the meat.

Handle turkey and chicken leftovers safely by cutting the meat off the bones within two hours of cooking it. Refrigerate the stuffing and the meat separately in shallow containers. Use leftover poultry and stuffing within three to four days.

Ground Beef
Like all red meats, beef is a nutrient-dense food, rich in protein, vitamin B_{12}, iron, and zinc. Grinding exposes more of the meat surface to bacteria, which multiply rapidly between 40° F. and 140° F. Ground beef is particularly susceptible to contamination from the bacterium *E. coli*. Cooked beef can also be contaminated from raw meat juices.

To keep bacterial levels low, refrigerate ground beef at 40° F. or less, and use within two days. To destroy bacteria, cook ground beef to at least 160° F.

Pork
Today's pork is about 50 percent leaner than it was just twenty-five years ago. Pork is also a nutrient-dense food, rich in thiamin, pantothenic acid, vitamin B_{12}, chromium, and iron. Like beef, lamb, and veal, pork is considered a "red meat," and is a very good nutritional buy.

When storing raw pork, put it in a plastic bag to avoid contaminating other cooked foods or produce. Keep it refrigerated at 40° F. and cook it within three to five days, or freeze it. For best quality, use frozen pork within three months, and defrost in the refrigerator, in cold water, or in the microwave. Fresh pork liver and convenience meals containing pork should be used within one to two days.

Pork must be adequately cooked to eliminate any disease-causing parasites and bacteria that may be present. It is still possible to contract trichinosis (caused by the parasite *Trichinella spiralis*) by eating undercooked pork, although the risk has been greatly reduced in recent years as compared to early last century. In addition, other food-borne microorganisms, such as *Salmonella, Staphylococcus aureus,* and *Listeria monocytogenes,* can be found in pork. These microorganisms are destroyed when pork is cooked to an internal temperature of 160° F.

Eggs

Eggs are one of nature's most complete foods. Rich sources of protein, vitamins A, B_6, B_7, B_{12}, and D, as well as iron, phosphorus, and zinc, eggs are one of the most nutrient dense yet inexpensive foods you can buy. But fresh eggs may contain *Salmonella* bacteria, which can cause a severe infection within four to seven days and can lead to severe or even fatal illness.

To avoid illness from eggs, only buy eggs kept in a refrigerator or refrigerator case. Avoid eggs sold from a cooler, since they may not have been kept sufficiently cold to prevent bacterial growth. Before buying, open the carton and make sure the eggs are clean and unbroken. Refrigerate them as soon as possible after purchase, in their original carton, and use them within four to five weeks. Use hard-boiled eggs (in the shell or peeled) within one week after cooking.

Wash hands, utensils, equipment, and work areas with hot, soapy water before and after they come in contact with raw eggs and egg-containing foods. Cook eggs until both the yolk and white are firm. Avoid fried and soft-boiled eggs unless the yolk is cooked to a firm consistency. Scrambled eggs should not be runny, and casseroles and other dishes containing eggs should be cooked to 160° F. Serve cooked eggs and egg-containing foods immediately after cooking.

For buffet-style serving, hot egg dishes should be kept hot, and cold egg dishes kept cold. Eggs and egg dishes such as quiches and soufflés may be refrigerated for serving later, but should be thoroughly reheated to 165° F. before serving. Cooked eggs, including hard-boiled eggs and egg-containing foods, should not remain unrefrigerated for more than two hours. If you cannot either reheat or refrigerate them within that time frame, throw them out. Leftover egg dishes that are promptly refrigerated can be kept for three to four days.

Oysters

Oysters are rich sources of many nutrients, including vitamin B_{12}, iodine, selenium, iron, and zinc. But raw oysters should never be eaten, most especially when you're pregnant. *Vibrio vulnificus* is a type of bacteria that occurs naturally in marine waters and is commonly found in Gulf of Mexico oysters. Within two days of consumption, this bacteria can cause chills, fever, nausea, and vomiting—and 40 percent of *Vibrio vulnificus* infections from raw oysters are fatal. The bacteria are not a result of pollution, so eating oysters from "clean" waters, or from reputable restaurants, does not provide protection.

Fortunately, fully cooking oysters completely kills the harmful bacteria. This way, you can safely enjoy them even during your pregnancy.

Dry Sausages

These types of sausages are not cooked, but use fermentation by lactic acid for preservation and for a distinctive flavor. The ingredients are mixed with spices and curing materials, put into casings, and submitted to an air-drying process. Dry sausages include chorizo; Frizzes; pepperoni; Lola, Lolita, and Lyons sausage; and Genoa salami. Because dry sausages are not cooked, the bacterium *E. coli* can survive the process of dry fermenting.

Currently, the USDA is looking into ways to overcome this problem. But until it can be solved, *pregnant women should not eat dry sausages.*

Cheeses

Hard cheeses such as cheddar, Swiss, and Parmesan are generally safe during pregnancy, as are the cooked soft cheeses like mozzarella on pizza. Certain soft cheeses, however, can become contaminated with bacteria called *Listeria*. Risky types include Mexican-style soft cheeses (queso blanco, queso fresco, queso de hoja, queso de crema, and asadero), feta cheese, brie, Camembert, and blue-veined cheeses (like Roquefort).

Symptoms of *Listeria* infection can develop from two to thirty days after you eat a contaminated food. If the infection spreads to your unborn baby, you could experience premature labor. Tell your doctor right away if you get any of these symptoms: fever and chills or other flulike symptoms; headache; nausea; vomiting.

Although *Listeria* is destroyed during cooking, it can grow in the refrigerator and survive in the freezer. To prevent infection, the FDA suggests the following precautions:

- Use hard cheeses, like cheddar, instead of soft cheeses during pregnancy.
- If you do use soft cheeses, cook them until they are bubbling.
- Use only pasteurized dairy products (stated on the label).
- If you do eat hard cheeses made from unpasteurized milk, use only those marked "aged sixty days" or longer.

Food for Thought: Your Health Now and Later

Besides wanting you to have a healthy child, I want *you* to be as healthy as possible. The Food for Thought sections at the end of certain chapters describe how the nutrients your unborn baby needs will also benefit your own health, now and for many years to come.

For instance, the whole grains, fiber, and magnesium that protect your baby from a future of diabetes also reduce your own risk of the disease. The Iowa Women's Health Study, which followed nearly 36,000 women for six years, reported the following[21]:

- Women who ate more than seventeen servings of whole grains per week, and those who ate more than twenty-four grams of fiber per day, reduced their risk of diabetes by 20 percent.
- Women who got at least 332 mg of magnesium per day reduced their risk of diabetes by 33 percent.

Likewise, the folic acid that is vital to your unborn baby's neurological development also protects you in three important ways:

- A recent study of more than 88,000 women found that, among those with a daily intake of 400 mcg of folic acid, the risk of developing colon cancer was reduced by 75 percent.
- The risk of coronary heart disease was reduced by nearly one-half among women who took a multivitamin daily, particularly if it contained folic acid and vitamin B_{12}, according to data from the Nurses' Health Study, a longitudinal study of more than 80,000 U.S. nurses[22]. In a study of more than 5,000 Canadian men and women aged 35 to 79, low levels of folic acid in the blood were associated with a 67 percent increased risk of death from coronary heart disease[23].
- Inadequate levels of folic acid and vitamin B_{12} and high levels of homocysteine in the blood may play roles in the development of Alzheimer's disease and senile dementia[24].

Menu Ideas for These Months

To make it easy to program your baby for good health, I've translated the dietary guidelines into menu suggestions, each specifically targeted toward women at a certain stage of pregnancy. I've also included lots of delicious recipes (indicated with an asterisk in the menu listings) that are designed to meet particular dietary needs of expectant mothers. If you're already pregnant, be sure to check out the menus and recipes for the first trimester (in Chapter 5), the second trimester (in Chapter 6), and the third trimester (in Chapter 7).

Menus for Before You Get Pregnant

FOCUS ON FOLIC ACID AND IRON

It is important to include ample amounts of folic acid and other B vitamins in your diet every day to reduce your baby's risk of congenital anomalies. These vital nutrients also help safeguard your own health. It is also important to get enough iron during these months, as most women have little or no iron stores when they do get pregnant, and iron-deficiency anemia can increase your risk of pregnancy complications.

The richest sources of folic acid (also called folate) and other B vitamins include asparagus, avocados, bananas, beans and lentils, whole-wheat bread, broccoli, chickpeas, oranges, spinach, and wheat germ. The richest sources of iron include beef, pork, poultry, seafood, eggs, nuts, spinach, broccoli, tomatoes, and wheat germ.

An asterisk after a menu item indicates a recipe that can be found at the end of this book.

BREAKFAST IDEAS
- Whole-wheat toast with peanut butter
- Vanilla yogurt with walnuts and wheat germ
- Chicken salad with raisins and grapes
- Hash Browns Supreme*
- Daybreak Date Bread* with sliced cheddar cheese
- Vegetable Quiche* with Pumpkin Raisin Nut Muffins*
- Wholesome Apple-Raisin Muffins* with hard-boiled eggs
- Banana-Orange Oatmeal Muffins* with milk

LUNCH OR DINNER IDEAS
- Beef and Tomato Tacos*
- Barbara's Meat Loaf* with baked potatoes and peas
- Southwest Salad*
- Cherry Glazed Pork Chops* with Deluxe Green Beans*
- Sunday Pot Roast* with steamed spinach
- Linguine with clam sauce
- Sweet and Sour Pork* with steamed rice
- Asian Chicken Salad*

SNACK IDEAS
- Rice pudding with dried cherries
- Tabouli or hummus on sesame crispbread
- Fruit salad with cheese crackers
- Sunrise Muffins* with milk

◄ *If you're planning to get pregnant* and are overweight, it would be wise to bring your weight down into the normal range before you start trying to conceive. To help you lose weight steadily and safely, I've devised a week's worth of menus for this 1,200-Calorie Reducing Diet Plan.

1,200-CALORIE REDUCING DIET PLAN

Breakfast	Lunch	Snack	Dinner

Whole-grain cereal
Fresh blueberries
Lowfat milk
Decaffeinated
  coffee
	Cottage cheese
	Hard-boiled egg
	Mixed greens
	Carrots and
	  cucumbers
	Sparkling water
		Graham crackers
		Lowfat milk
			Grilled
			  hamburger
			Corn on the
			  cob
			Mixed salad
			  and dressing
			Fresh
			  strawberries
			Iced tea

Bran cereal
Raisins
Lowfat milk
Decaffeinated
  coffee
	Peanut butter and
	  mango sandwich
	  on whole-wheat
	  bread
	Fresh apple
	Iced tea
		Lowfat yogurt
		Banana
			Baked flounder
			Baked sweet
			  potato
			Steamed
			  broccoli
			Iced coffee

Lowfat yogurt
Wheat germ
Fresh strawberries
Decaffeinated
  coffee
	Chef salad
	  with 1 oz. each
	  ham, cheese,
	  chicken
	Mixed greens with
	  croutons
	Iced tea
		Frozen yogurt	Roasted turkey
			Winter squash
			Steamed rice
			Sparkling
			  water

Hot oatmeal
Grated cheddar
  cheese
Cantaloupe
  melon balls
Decaffeinated
  coffee
	Tuna sandwich with
	  lettuce and
	  tomato on
	  toasted rye, mayo
	Sparkling water
		Lowfat milk
		Graham crackers
			Two-egg
			  omelet with
			  bean sprouts
			  and spring
			  onions
			Steamed rice
			Hot tea

Breakfast	Lunch	Snack	Dinner
Cracked wheat toast	Clam chowder made with lowfat milk	Frozen yogurt	Pasta with marinara
Farmer cheese	Oyster crackers		Mushroom and spinach salad
Fresh grapefruit	Iced tea		
Decaffeinated coffee			Iced tea
Grilled sandwich with lowfat cheese	Ham sandwich with lettuce and tomato on toasted raisin bread	Lowfat yogurt Graham crackers	Baked pork chops
Fresh orange juice			Baked apple
Decaffeinated coffee	Sparkling water		Wild rice
			Peas and carrots
			Hot tea
Hard-boiled egg	Roast beef sandwich on whole-wheat bread with lowfat cheese	Fresh plums	Chicken stir-fry with Chinese vegetables
Toasted oatmeal bread slices		Lowfat cheese	
Tomato juice			Steamed rice
Decaffeinated coffee	Iced tea		Hot tea

3 ❧ FOUNDATIONS FOR A HEALTHY PREGNANCY

Important as prenatal nutrition is, it does not tell the whole story when it comes to metabolic programming. Many other factors also strongly influence your unborn baby's growth and development. To strengthen the foundations for a healthy pregnancy, and positively affect your child's lifelong well-being, you need to protect your own health and conscientiously avoid harmful substances.

The majority of the advice presented in this chapter applies to all expectant mothers, from the first day of pregnancy to the last. In addition, each section ends with special suggestions for women who are not yet pregnant but who hope to conceive soon.

Your Health Status: Why It Matters

From your level of fitness to your age to your medical history, the health status of your own body is a major determining factor for your child's future health. Here's what you need to know and do to prepare your body for the healthiest pregnancy possible.

YOUR PHYSICAL FITNESS

Years ago, females were treated like delicate flowers. Organized sports for girls were practically unheard of, high school students were excused from gym class during menstruation, and expectant mothers were cautioned against the slightest exertion.

Today the philosophy of women's fitness is dramatically different. Strong women are seen as beautiful, female athletes are admired, and physical fitness has become an important goal for women of all ages. Pregnant women who are physically fit enjoy added advantages: They tend to sleep better and feel less fatigued during pregnancy, and after delivery they generally are quicker to regain their energy and their figures.

If you had been exercising regularly before you conceived, and yours is not a high-risk pregnancy, your doctor will probably give you the go-ahead to keep working out. Moderation, though, is key. Even if your fitness level is excellent, it's best to reduce the intensity and length of your workouts. If you are accustomed to doing an intense aerobic or weight-lifting workout, it may be advisable to switch to a different type of exercise. Walking and swimming are the two types of exercise that are most beneficial during pregnancy because they are least likely to challenge your balance or restrict blood flow to the uterus. (For more information, see Chapter 6.)

◄ *If you're planning to get pregnant,* and have not been working out regularly, *now is not the time to take up an ambitious exercise regimen.* Instead, get your doctor's okay for a moderate level of activity, such as walking for twenty minutes three times a week. If you are an avid exerciser, consider cutting back on the intensity and frequency of your workouts. Extreme physical activity can impair your fertility by interfering with ovulation.

YOUR AGE

Over the past twenty-five years, there has been a significant increase in the age at which many women have children. Women today are often pursuing higher education and careers during the ages when their mothers and grandmothers were having babies. For example, nowadays a woman who is thirty years old or older is four times more likely to be having her first child as compared to a woman of the same age in 1975. Women of thirty-five and older are seven times more likely to become mothers now than they would have been twenty-five years ago. And for women forty years of age and up, today's pregnancy rate is ten times higher than it was a generation ago.

Healthy women over thirty-five who follow the prenatal recommendations of their healthcare providers have nearly as good a chance of delivering a healthy baby as do younger women. Age does carry some additional risks, however. An older mother is more likely to have a preexisting health condition that could affect her pregnancy. She is also at higher risk for having a baby with certain genetic birth defects, such as Down's syndrome.

If you are over age 35, it is especially important that you obtain early prenatal care. Your doctor also may suggest that you undergo diagnostic testing, such as amniocentesis, early in your pregnancy. (See Chapter 4 for more information.)

◄ *If you're planning to get pregnant,* understand that fertility naturally drops as a woman's age increases. If you've been trying without success to conceive, ask your doctor about the advisability of infertility testing and treatment.

IMMUNIZATIONS

Pregnancy is no time to get sick. Check with your doctor to make sure that you're up to date on all immunizations, including the following:

- tetanus (with a booster received within the last ten years)
- diphtheria (with a booster received within the last ten years)
- measles/mumps/rubella (the vaccine is given once, usually in childhood)
- hepatitis B (particularly if you work in the healthcare field, where your risk of exposure is higher)
- influenza (especially if you have asthma or another chronic respiratory condition)

If your medical records show that you are not current on all your immunizations and you're already pregnant, ask your doctor what steps you should take to minimize your risk of contracting these diseases. Vaccinations that are prepared with live viruses (measles, mumps, rubella, yellow fever) should not be given during pregnancy. Other vaccinations (influenza, diphtheria, polio, tetanus, rabies), while not routinely given during pregnancy, can be used with little risk after the first trimester. Therefore, your doctor may advise that you be vaccinated if you come in contact with someone with the disease or, in the case of tetanus, if you receive a wound.

Rubella, also known as German measles, warrants your particular attention because when this disease is contracted during early pregnancy, it can cause birth defects. If you have been vaccinated or have already had this disease, you are immune. But if a blood test reveals that you are *not* immune to rubella and you are already pregnant, follow your doctor's advice for avoiding contact with anyone who may have this contagious disease.

◄ *If you're planning to get pregnant,* and are not immune to rubella, get your vaccination as soon as possible. Then wait two or three months before trying to conceive. This is also the time to catch up on any other vaccinations you may be missing.

PREEXISTING MEDICAL CONDITIONS

Make sure your obstetrician is fully aware of any medical conditions you may have. Some chronic diseases require specialized prenatal care, and certain medications should be avoided during pregnancy.

Diabetes

If you have diabetes, it's vital that you maintain good blood glucose control throughout your pregnancy, so you'll need to work closely with your diabetes healthcare team. Without proper blood glucose control, a diabetic woman is at increased risk for having a baby with birth defects, and may also experience immediate and long-term health problems herself.

◄ *If you're planning to get pregnant,* tell your doctor well in advance. The risk of birth defects in babies born to diabetic mothers decreases most significantly when the disease is well controlled prior to conception and in the early weeks of pregnancy.

Phenylketonuria

For the past forty years, all newborns in the United States have been screened at birth for phenylketonuria (PKU), a genetic disorder of amino acid metabolism that leads to mental retardation. If you were treated for PKU, which includes a special diet until about age 6, it is important for you to have diet therapy again. Otherwise, high levels of phenylalanine may cause birth defects and mental retardation in your developing baby.

◄ *If you're planning to get pregnant,* begin now to work with your medical doctor and registered dietitian to lower your blood levels of phenylalanine. Diet therapy that begins before conception is most effective in reducing risks associated with PKU[1].

Infertility Treatments

If you underwent infertility treatments prior to your pregnancy, you may be in less than optimal nutritional shape. Fertility medications can result in bloating and nausea and interfere with appetite. Likewise, the emotional effects of infertility may sap the energy needed to plan for and prepare healthful meals. That's why it's especially important for former infertility patients to maintain good eating habits throughout pregnancy.

◄ *If you're planning to get pregnant* and are undergoing infertility treatments now, remember not to let your diet slip. By safeguarding your nutritional status, you can only improve your odds of conceiving.

Dental Problems

Dental problems are often an unrecognized source of infection, and infection can increase the risk for preterm birth. Fortunately, dental work is generally safe during pregnancy. Be sure your dentist knows that you are pregnant. If possible, postpone dental X rays until after your baby is born; otherwise, make sure your dentist provides you with a lead apron to protect your unborn baby from the X rays.

◄ *If you're planning to get pregnant,* understand that infection can undermine your ability to conceive. If you've been postponing any fillings, crowns, or other dental work, take care of these problems now, before you start trying to conceive.

SCREENING TESTS

It is important to be screened for diseases that could affect your unborn baby, such as sexually transmitted diseases, HIV, and tuberculosis. Depending on your ethnic background, you and your partner also may be tested for inheritable diseases such as Tay-Sachs disease, sickle-cell disease, and thalassemia. Your doctor can give you complete information about such screening tests.

◄ *If you're planning to get pregnant,* you have the advantage of being screened before you actually conceive. It's wise for your partner to be tested now, too.

MEDICATIONS

While many drugs can be used safely during pregnancy, others must be avoided entirely in order to prevent serious harm to the unborn baby. Be sure that each one of your healthcare providers—not just your obstetrician, but also your allergist, internist, dentist, and so on—knows that you are pregnant. That information is crucial in determining whether or not the benefits outweigh the risks in prescribing any particular medication.

With your doctors, review the list of every prescription and over-the-counter medication you currently take, whether you take it regularly or not. If you have a chronic condition such as allergies, your doctor may switch you from one type of medication to another type that is safer during pregnancy. Do not, however, suddenly stop taking important medications, such as those for asthma or seizures, without your doctor's approval.

Certain medications are most risky in the early stages of pregnancy, while others are harmful later in pregnancy. Table 3-1 summarizes, by trimester, the medications that may be dangerous to your unborn baby.

◄ *If you're planning to get pregnant,* be sure to tell your doctor you are trying to conceive. He or she may advise you to stop taking particular medications *before* you start trying to become pregnant. If your doctor wants you to start a new medication, be sure to ask whether it can interfere with fertility or is dangerous to a fetus. If you have been using birth control pills, be aware that most

TABLE 3-1. DRUGS THAT MAY ADVERSELY
AFFECT THE FETUS AND THE NEWBORN INFANT

Drugs that *probably* cause adverse effects when taken during the *first trimester*

Aminopterin
Anticonvulsants
  Acetazolamide (Diamox)
  Carbamazepine (Tegretol)
  Clonazepam (Klonopin)
  Clorazepate (Tranxene)
  Diazepam (Valium)
  Ethosuximide (Zarontin)
  Felbamate (Felbatol)
  Gabapentin (Neurontin)
  Lamotrigine (Lamictal)
  Mephenytoin (Mesantoin)
  Methsuximide (Celontin)
  Paramethadione (Paradione)
  Phenacemide (Phenurone)
  Phenobarbital (Luminal)
  Phensuximide (Milontin)
  Phenytoin (Dilantin)
  Primidone (Mysoline)
  Topiramate (Topamax)
  Trimethadione (Tridione)
  Valproic acid (Depakene)
Antithyroid drugs
Cytarabine
Danazol
Diethylstilbestrol
Ethanol
Etretinate
Finasteride
Fluorouracil

HMG-CoA reductase inhibitors
  Atorvastatin (Lipitor)
  Cerivastatin (Baycol)
  Fluvastin (Lescol)
  Lovastatin (Mevacor)
  Pravastatin (Pravachol)
  Simvastatin (Zocor)
Iodides
Isotretinoin
Kanamycin
Mercaptopurine
Methotrexate
Misoprostol
Opioid analgesics
  Alfentanil (Alfenta)
  Codeine
  Fentanyl (Actiq, Sublimaze, Duragesic)
  Hydrocodone (Dilaudid)
  Levorphanol (Levo-Dromoran)
  Meperidine (Demerol)
  Methadone (Dolophine)
  Morphine
  Oxycodone (OxyContin, Roxicodone)
  Oxymorphone (Numorphan)
  Propoxyphene (Darvon)
  Sufentanil (Sufenta)
Progestins (female sex hormones)
  Ethynodiol

Hydroxyprogesterone
Medroxyprogesterone
Megestrol (Megace)
Norethindrone
Norgestrel (Ovrette)
Progesterone

Quinine
Streptomycin
Testosterone
Warfarin

Drugs that *possibly* cause adverse effects when taken during the *first* trimester

Angiotensin-converting enzyme
  inhibitors
  Candesartan (Atacand)
  Eprosartan (Teveten)
  Iosartan (Cozaar)
  Irbesartan (Avapro)
  Irbesartan hydrochlorothiazide
  Valsartan (Diovan)
Busulfan
Chlorambucil
Estrogens (female sex hormones)
  Chlorotrianisene (Tace)
  Diethylstilbestrol
  Estradiol (Estrace, Estraderm)
  Estrogens, conjugated
    (Premarin)
  Estrogens, esterified (Estratab,
    Menest)
  Estrone

Estropipate (Ogen)
Ethinyl estradiol (Estinyl)
Quinestrol (Estrovis)
Lithium
Mebendazole
Monoamine oxidase inhibitors
  Isocarboxazid (Marplan)
  Phenelzine (Nardil)
  Tranylcypromine (Parnate)
Oral contraceptives
Piperazine
Rifampin
Tetracyclines
  Demeclocycline (Declomycin)
  Doxycycline (Vibramycin)
  Methacycline (Rondomycin)
  Minocycline (Minocin)
  Oxytetracycline (Terramycin)
  Tetracycline (Achromycin V)

Drugs that *probably* cause adverse effects when taken during the *second* and *third* trimesters

Amiodarone
Androgens (male sex hormones)
  Fluoxymesterone
  Methyltestosterone
  Testosterone

Angiotensin-converting enzyme
  inhibitors
  Candesartan (Atacand)
  Eprosartan (Teveten)
  Iosartan (Cozaar)

Irbesartan (Avapro)
Irbesartan hydrochlorothiazide
Valsartan (Diovan)
Antithyroid drugs
Aspirin
Benzodiazepines
  Alprazolam (Xanax)
  Bromazepam (Lectopam)
  Chlordiazepoxide (Librium)
  Clonazepam (Klonopin)
  Clorazepate (Tranxene)
  Dazepam (Valim, Vazepam)
  Flurazepam (Dalmane)
  Halazepam (Paxipam)
  Ketazolam (Loftran)
  Lorazepam (Ativan)
  Midazolam (Versed)
  Nitrazepam (Mogadon)
  Oxazepam (Serax)
  Prazepam (Centrax)
  Quazepam (Doral)
  Temazepam (Restoril)
  Triazolam (Halcion)
Chloramphenicol
Estrogens
  Chlorotrianisene (Tace)
  Diethylstilbestrol
  Estradiol (Estrace, Estraderm)
  Estrogens, conjugated
    (Premarin)
  Estrogens, esterified (Estratab,
    Menest)
  Estrone
  Estropipate (Ogen)
  Ethinyl estradiol (Estinyl)
  Quinestrol (Estrovis)

Ethanol
Finasteride
HMG-CoA reductase inhibitors
  Atorvastatin (Lipitor)
  Cerivastatin (Baycol)
  Fluvastatin (Lescol)
  Lovastatin (Mevacor)
  Pravastatin (Pravachol)
  Simvastatin (Zocor)
Iodides
Kanamycin
Lithium
Nonsteroidal anti-inflammatory
  drugs
Opioid analgesics
  Alfentanil (Alfenta)
  Codeine
  Fentanyl (Actiq, Sublimaze,
    Duragesic)
  Hydrocodone (Dilaudid)
  Levorphanol (Levo-Dromoran)
  Meperidine (Demerol)
  Methadone (Dolophine)
  Morphine
  Oxycodone (OxyContin,
    Roxicodone)
  Oxymorphone (Numorphan)
  Propoxyphene (Darvon)
  Sufentanil (Sufenta)
Phenothiazine
  Acetophenazine (Tindal)
  Chlorpromazine (Thorazine)
  Fluphenazine (Permitil, Prolixin)
  Mesoridazine (Serentil)
  Perphenazine (Trilafon)
  Prochlorperazine (Compazine)

Promazine (Sparine)
Thioridazine (Mellaril)
Trifluoperazine (Stelazine)
Triflupromazine (Vesprin)
Progestins (female sex hormones)
Ethynodiol
Hydroxyprogesterone
Medroxyprogesterone
Megestrol (Megace)
Norethindrone
Norgestrel (Ovrette)
Progesterone
Rifampin
Streptomycin
Sulfonamides (anti-infectives)
Multiple sulfonamides (Triple Sulfa No.2)
Sulfacytine (Renoquid)
Sulfadiazine
Sulfamethizole (Thiosulfil)
Sulfamethoxazole (Gantanol)
Sulfasalazine (Azulfidine)
Sulfisoxazole (Gantrisin)
Sulfonylureas (oral antidiabetic drugs)
Acetohexamide (Dymelor)
Chlorpropamide (Diabinese)
Glimepiride (Amaryl)
Glipizide (Glucotrol)
Glyburide (DiaBeta, Micronase)
Tolazamide (Tolamide, Tolinase)
Tolbutamide (Orinase)

Tetracyclines
Demeclocycline (Declomycin)
Doxycycline (Vibramycin)
Methacycline (Rondomycin)
Minocycline (Minocin)
Oxytetracycline (Terramycin)
Tetracycline (Achromycin V)
Thiazide diuretics
Bendroflumethiazide (Naturetin)
Benzthiazide (Aquatag, Marazide)
Chlorothiazide (Diruil)
Cyclothiazide (Anhydron)
Hydrochlorothiazide (Esidrix, Hydrodiuril)
Hydroflumethiazide (Diucardin, Saluron)
Methyclothiazide (Enduron)
Polythiazide (Renese)
Trichlormethiazide (Metahydrin, Naqua)
Tricyclic antidepressants
Amitriptyline (Elavil)
Amoxapine (Asendin)
Clomipramine (Anafranil)
Desipramine (Norpramin)
Doxepin (Adapin, Sinequan)
Imipramine (Trofanil)
Nortriptyline (Aventyl, Pamelor)
Protriptyline (Vivactil)
Trimipramine (Surmontil)
Warfarin

Drugs that *possibly* cause effects when taken during the *second and third trimesters*

Acetazolamide

Clemastine

Diphenhydramine

Ethacrynic acid

Fluoroquinolones (anti-infectives)

  Ciprofloxacin (Cipro)

  Grepafloxacin (Raxar)

  Levofloxacin (Levaquin)

Lomefloxacin (Maxaquin)

Norfloxacin (Noroxin)

Ofloxacin (Floxin)

Sparfloxacin (Zagam)

Trovafloxacin (Trovan)

Haloperidol

Hydroxyzine

Promethazine

Adapted from Table 1, *The Essential Guide to Prescription Drugs 2000,* by J. J. Rybacki and J. W. Long. New York: HarperCollins, 1999, p. 1119. Used with permission.

doctors suggest you stop using them at least three months before you try to conceive.

Toxins and Your Unborn Baby

Nearly everything a pregnant woman breathes, touches, or ingests has the potential to affect her unborn baby's metabolic programming. Some substances deserve only a word of caution, while others are so damaging that they must be scrupulously avoided.

SMOKING: EVERY PUFF A DANGER

If you are a smoker, you're not alone. In the United States, approximately 46 million people smoke regularly. That means nearly one in four men and one in five women—including one in eight expectant mothers—are smokers[2].

No doubt you've heard about the health dangers smokers face: heart disease, stroke, emphysema, lung cancer, cervical cancer. But have you also heard how harmful cigarettes are to your unborn baby? For instance:

- Miscarriages are more common among smokers[3].
- Congenital malformations occur more frequently among babies born to smokers[4].
- With each cigarette, you expose your unborn baby to thousands of toxic substances, including the poisons carbon monoxide and cyanide. Your body must divert essential nutrients to detoxify these substances, thereby reducing the amount of these nutrients available for fetal growth.
- Carbon monoxide also binds to hemoglobin and lowers the amount of oxygen in your blood. This, in turn, reduces the amount of oxygen to the placenta, the vital middleman in your baby's growth and development. The result is an increase in placental infarcts, or areas where the placental tissue dies due to lack of oxygen. This is one reason why smokers' babies tend to be much smaller at birth.
- Smoking causes a unique kind of malnutrition, resulting in babies with not only lower birthweights, but also smaller head circumferences and shorter lengths[5]. As you will read about in Chapter 4, these are termed "symmetrically small babies," a condition associated with various health problems.
- Expectant mothers who smoke are far more likely to deliver prematurely[6]. In fact, studies suggest that as many as 27 percent of all premature deliveries in this country are related to smoking[7].

Nor does the danger to your child cease the day he or she is born. The evidence:

- A child exposed to tobacco in the womb may later show impaired neurological development[8].
- Babies born to smokers are at increased risk for sudden infant death syndrome (SIDS)[9].

- Smoking by either parent during pregnancy is associated with a higher risk for childhood cancer for the baby[10].
- Among symmetrically small babies, growth continues to be slow during the first postnatal year.
- Symmetrically small babies are also at increased risk for developing hypertension later in life.

It's fortunate, then, that exposure to cigarette smoke is one factor of this pregnancy that's entirely under your control. So if you smoke, please quit now, if not for your own sake, then for the good of your unborn child. "For years, I had smoked two packs a day. But once I got pregnant, I knew I had to stop," says Annemarie, a mother of three. "When I craved a smoke, it helped to chew gum, suck on hard candy, or just keep busy. Mostly it was a question of willpower." If you need help quitting, ask your doctor or contact a support group. The nicotine patch appears to be safe in pregnancy, and is certainly much safer than smoking[11].

If you've already quit, or never did smoke, good for you! Remember, though, to avoid secondhand smoke. Just being around smokers while you're pregnant can significantly increase your risk of having a baby who's born small for his or her gestational age[12]. Janna, a mother of four, says, "When I was pregnant, the smell of cigarettes made me nauseous. I didn't let people smoke in my house, car, or office. Walking down the street, I'd cross to the other side if someone near me was smoking. And if I couldn't get a table in the nonsmoking section of a restaurant, I'd just leave. No fancy meal was worth risking my baby's health."

If your partner is a smoker, encourage him to quit in support of you and your unborn child. At the very least, he should carefully avoid smoking in your home and in your presence. Says Annemarie, "When I was pregnant, my husband would never smoke around me. We both knew the secondhand smoke would be bad for the baby. Also, since it had been hard for me to quit smoking, he wanted to help me avoid temptation."

◄ *If you're planning to get pregnant,* realize that smoking can undermine a woman's ability to conceive[13]. Cigarettes also siphon off important nutrients, compromising your nutritional status. Since you certainly won't want to be smoking once you are pregnant, the wisest course of action is to quit right now.

THE DEVASTATING EFFECTS OF ALCOHOL

The link between birth defects and drinking during pregnancy has been recognized since early Greek civilization, when newly married couples were forbidden by law to drink alcohol. Throughout medical history, pregnant women have been warned to abstain from alcohol because of its potential to cause harm to the developing baby. Yet it wasn't until 1968, when French scientists identified a specific array of congenital malformations of the face and mental retardation that were associated with drinking during pregnancy, that scientific evidence finally supported the age-old folk advice to abstain from alcohol during pregnancy[14].

By 1971, the condition became known as fetal alcohol syndrome (FAS). In the United States, FAS affects approximately five thousand babies per year—that's one in every seven hundred births—making it the leading cause of mental retardation and learning and behavioral problems[15,16].

More than 80 percent of children with FAS suffer the following:

• delayed growth, both before and after birth
• mental retardation
• poor coordination
• attention deficit disorder with hyperactivity (ADHD)
• malformations of the face

Additionally, 20 to 50 percent of FAS children have these problems:

- birth defects of various kinds
- cardiac problems
- impaired vision
- hearing loss

The more a woman drinks, the more profoundly affected her baby is likely to be. FAS occurs in 30 to 40 percent of babies born to women who are alcoholics or chronic alcohol abusers (defined as drinking six or more drinks per day) throughout pregnancy.

Yet even when a woman's alcohol consumption is significantly less than this, her baby is still at risk. In the United States, nearly fifty thousand babies—that's one in seventy babies—are born each year with a condition called fetal alcohol effects. This condition is characterized by some, but not all, of the birth defects associated with FAS. Even moderate drinking—as little as three drinks per week—more than doubles your baby's risk for being born weighing less than five and a half pounds[17].

This means that when you are pregnant, total abstinence is the only prudent course. *There is no safe amount of alcohol that you can consume during pregnancy.*

Alcohol is poison to your unborn baby for several reasons:

- Alcohol can alter levels of at least seven vital nutrients. These nutritional deficits contribute to an increase in birth defects.
- The amniotic fluid surrounding the fetus acts as a reservoir for alcohol. Because the baby lacks the necessary enzymes to metabolize alcohol, he is exposed to it long after your body has cleared it from your own blood supply.
- Alcohol interferes with protein synthesis, a critical process in your baby's development. Potential consequences for the unborn baby include stunted growth, birth defects, and mental retardation.
- Alcohol also may be directly toxic to the placenta, causing the unborn baby to suffer a special kind of malnutrition.

Despite official advisories first issued in 1981 warning against the use of alcohol by pregnant women and women considering becoming pregnant, too many women do continue to drink while pregnant. In fact, according to a national survey by the Centers for Disease Control, drinking during pregnancy is on the rise[18,19,20]. Between 1991 and 1995, the number of pregnant women who reported any drinking increased from 12.4 percent to 16.3 percent; women drinking five or more drinks on occasion increased from 0.7 percent to 2.9 percent; and expectant mothers who consumed seven or more drinks per week increased from 0.8 percent to 3.5 percent. This is an extremely dangerous trend.

If you cannot stop drinking, tell your doctor at once. You have a medical problem, and medical treatment is available. Fortunately, many pregnant women find it easy to stop drinking because they develop an aversion to alcohol. "Alcohol did not appeal to me when I was expecting. The smell, the taste, the very thought of it turned me off. Maybe it was Mother Nature's way of saying I didn't need this," reports Abigail, a mother of three.

◄ *If you're planning to get pregnant,* understand that alcohol's harmful effects begin even before you conceive. Heavy or chronic drinking can be an underlying cause of infertility for both sexes. In women, it can lead to irregular menstrual cycles and can prevent ovulation. In men, alcohol can lower the male hormone testosterone, leading to low sperm counts. Alcohol also depletes your system of vital nutrients. When you're trying to get pregnant, the safest course of action is not to drink at all, or at least to limit your consumption to no more than one or two drinks per week.

CAFFEINE: IS IT OKAY?

The majority of research on caffeine and pregnancy has shown that moderate consumption—about one cup of coffee a day—is probably safe. Some studies, however, have reported that caffeine consumption is associated with an increased risk for miscarriage, fetal growth retardation, and premature rupture of membranes (when the amniotic sac breaks prior to thirty-seven weeks' gestation)[21,22,23,24,25].

There are several factors that make caffeine problematic:

- It's addictive (which is why you can get withdrawal headaches when you skip your usual cup).
- Caffeine affects the central nervous system (which is why it wakes you up).
- It acts as a diuretic, which can contribute to dehydration; in turn, dehydration can trigger preterm uterine contractions.
- Caffeine can interfere with the absorption of minerals, particularly calcium, which your unborn baby needs in order to grow properly.

The Food and Drug Administration advises pregnant women to consume caffeine only in moderation. Better yet, switch to decaffeinated coffee.

What about tea? Some teas do contain significant amounts of caffeine, so select a decaffeinated brand, or choose teas made from only peppermint or ginger. Do not drink any tea or herbal preparation that contains comfrey, calcmus, pennyroyal, sassafras, or coltsfoot—all of which are carcinogenic.

"I used to drink three cups of coffee each day, plus a fair amount of tea," says Sharifa, a mother of two. "But as soon as I found out I was pregnant, I cut out coffee altogether, and had just one cup of tea in the morning. The smell of a fresh-brewed pot of java was tempting at first, but if I just put my hand on my belly and thought about my baby, the craving passed quickly. Pretty soon I didn't think about coffee at all."

◄ *If you're planning to get pregnant,* it would be wise to cut back on coffee or switch to decaffeinated, because some research suggests a link between caffeine and an increased risk of infertility. Helena, a mother of twins, recalls, "I had been in the habit of drinking five cups of coffee a day, so I decided to quit before trying to get pregnant. To minimize the headaches from caffeine withdrawal, I weaned myself gradually. Within three weeks, I was off of coffee completely. And a month later, I was pregnant!"

ENVIRONMENTAL TOXINS AND HOW TO AVOID THEM

Our modern environment is filled with chemicals and infectious agents that can have serious adverse effects on your unborn baby's growth and development. The key to preventing such problems is avoidance. Here's what you need to watch out for:

- Dry-cleaning solutions. Remove plastic wrap from dry-cleaned garments and allow them to air out before wearing.
- Pesticides. Limit the use of chemicals on your lawn and garden. Wash produce thoroughly before eating.
- Paints, solvents, and other household chemicals. Avoid touching these or breathing in their fumes. If you must use these chemicals, wear rubber gloves and make sure you have adequate ventilation.
- Lead. Check your water supply for lead content, particularly if you live in a home built before 1990, when lead solder was often used in home plumbing. Any level greater than fifteen parts per billion calls for treatment to reduce the lead in your water. Contact the Environmental Protection Agency (EPA) Safe Drinking Water Hotline at 800-426-4791 for a list of state-certified testing labs in your area.
- Cat feces. Cats can carry a parasite that causes toxoplasmosis. If a pregnant woman gets infected, her unborn baby may suffer brain damage, blindness, or even death[26,27]. So have someone else change your cat's litter box throughout your pregnancy. Avoid gardening in areas that outdoor cats might frequent, and always wear gloves whenever you do garden.
- Saunas and hot tubs. These should also be avoided, particularly

during the first trimester, because they can raise your internal body temperature to levels that may be harmful to your unborn baby.

Safeguarding Your Nutritional Status

We've learned a lot about how lifestyle choices and health concerns—from smoking and drinking to excessive exercise to illness and medications—can directly affect your unborn baby. But there's another aspect to consider as well: their potential to undermine your nutritional status. Table 3-2 shows how various lifestyle habits, chronic conditions, and medicines can deplete your body of the specific vitamins and minerals your growing baby needs. Let the information in this table provide one more motivating force to help you keep your baby's metabolic programming on a positive track.

For the sake of your unborn baby, you're taking better care of yourself than ever: You're eating right, shunning alcohol and cigarettes, and avoiding toxins of all types. That's good for both you and your baby, now and in the future. As you program your baby for lifelong well-being, you're also maximizing your own chances for long-term good health. You're more likely to be able to provide your child with your own loving and capable presence for many decades to come—and that's one of the most valuable gifts your child will ever receive.

TABLE 3-2. FACTORS THAT CAN UNDERMINE YOUR NUTRITIONAL STATUS

	VITAMINS									MINERALS					
	A	Thiamin	Riboflavin	Niacin	Pyridoxine	B_{12}	Folic Acid	C	D	Calcium	Copper	Iron	Magnesium	Potassium	Zinc
Lifestyle Habits															
Smoking	X					X	X	X						X	X
Alcohol use	X	X			X		X		X				X		X
Physical exercise			X												
Stress								X							
Chronic Conditions															
Diabetes								X							
Kidney stones					X										
Arthritis					X										
Medications															
Antacids							X			X	X				
Antibacterials			X	X	X		X		X	X					
Anti-cancer drugs							X						X		
Anticonvulsants							X		X						
Antihypertensives					X	X									
Anti-inflammatory							X		X			X			

Antimalarials

Diuretics

H2-Receptor antagonists

Hypocholesterolemics

Laxatives

Oral contraceptives

Steroids

Tranquilizers

Adapted from *Prevention's Healing with Vitamins* © 1996 by Rodale Press. Permission granted by Rodale Press, 400 S. Tenth St., Emmaus, PA 18098.

4 ❧ PRENATAL CARE
AND YOUR BABY'S GROWTH

The quality of prenatal care that you receive directly affects your unborn baby's metabolic programming. And that, in turn, will directly affect your child's health for his or her entire life. That's why it is so important to find a qualified healthcare provider you can trust. Then you'll need to schedule regular checkups, attend them all, and follow your doctor's instructions to the letter.

Most women choose an obstetrician, a physician who specializes in prenatal care. If yours is not a high-risk pregnancy, you may want to receive your prenatal care from a trusted family physician or an experienced midwife. However, if you are at risk for pregnancy complications (because you have a history of pregnancy problems or are expecting multiples, for example) your best choice is a maternal-fetal medicine specialist—an obstetrician who has received additional specialized training and put it to use in the management of high-risk pregnancies.

Your Doctor

Think of your obstetrician or other healthcare provider as your medical partner during your pregnancy. You are on a unique nine-month journey that will change your life forever. As partners, both of you have rights and responsibilities[1].

You have the right to:

- Get quality care without discrimination
- Privacy during your exams and confidentiality of your medical records
- Know the professional status of your healthcare providers and their fees
- Be advised of your condition, treatment, options, and the expected outcome
- Be actively involved in decisions about your care
- Refuse treatment
- Agree or refuse to participate in any research that affects your care

You have the responsibility to:

- Provide accurate and complete health information
- Let your healthcare providers know if you do not understand the medical procedures or what you are expected to do

The more information your doctor has about you and your pregnancy, the better prepared he or she is to detect and treat any potential health problems. If going to the doctor makes you nervous, you may not remember to discuss everything you should, so I've written out the most common questions your obstetrician may ask. Before your first prenatal checkup, get a journal or notebook and spend some time recording your answers to the questions below. This creates an overall picture of your past and current health, and helps your obstetrician plan the pregnancy care that's right for you and your unborn baby.

Your Family Health History

- Your and your partner's ethnic and racial backgrounds
- Inherited genetic disorders
- Any previous children born with a birth defect

Medical and Surgical History

- Current and past medications
- Allergies and allergic reactions
- Medical conditions
- Prior surgeries
- Exposure to infectious diseases

Menstrual History

- Your age at menarche (your first menstrual period)
- Date of your last menstrual period
- Use of birth control pills
- Other methods of contraception

Lifestyle Habits

- Your work, if employed
- Alcohol use
- Cigarette use
- Recreational drug use
- Exposure to toxic substances

Past Pregnancies

- Length of gestation (including pregnancy losses and sponta-neous or induced abortions)
- Complications before and after delivery
- Length of labor
- Method of delivery
- Condition of the newborn, including birthweight and compli-cations

WHAT YOUR DOCTOR NEEDS FROM YOU

Arrange to have your medical records from your other doctors (including your infertility specialist, if you have one) sent directly to your obstetrician, or bring them with you to your first prenatal appointment. This can save time and money since you will be able to avoid having to repeat many laboratory tests that may have already been done, such as hemoglobin and hematocrit tests to indicate the level of iron in your blood.

If this is not your first pregnancy, you should provide your obstetrician with complete information regarding prior pregnancies, whether they resulted in a birth or not. Research shows that there's a strong tendency to repeat the birthweight and gestational age at birth of previous pregnancies. If any of your pregnancies ended three or more weeks early, or if any of your children had a birthweight of less than 5½ pounds, your doctor needs to know. He or she will draw up a medical plan that will help to minimize the risk of experiencing such problems this time.

Also talk to your female relatives about their pregnancies, since genetics may play an important role in the course and outcome of your pregnancy. The risk of prematurity (defined as being born three or more weeks early) may be carried through the maternal side of the family tree. And premature babies are at significantly increased risk for a host of problems, including hearing loss, vision loss, respiratory disorders, serious developmental disabilities, even death. So ask your mother, sisters, and maternal aunts if their pregnancies ended earlier than expected, and if they encountered any other problems such as heavy bleeding with delivery. Armed with this knowledge, you can take extra precautions to reduce these family history risks.

Family history of a genetic disease is also vital information for your obstetrician. He or she may want to test both you and your partner to determine if either of you carries the genes for that disease.

WHAT YOU SHOULD EXPECT FROM YOUR DOCTOR

Your obstetrician should discuss the following issues with you and your partner:

- the type of care given in his or her office or clinic
- necessary laboratory tests
- the expected course of the pregnancy
- the timing of subsequent visits
- signs and symptoms you should report to the doctor, and actions you should take if they occur
- what to do if bleeding occurs
- what to do in case of emergency
- how to recognize labor and what to do when it begins
- what to do when your membranes rupture (your water breaks)
- plans for hospital admission
- labor and delivery
- analgesic and anesthetic options
- educational literature
- available childbirth and infant care classes
- tours of the newborn nursery, NICU, and labor and delivery unit

PRENATAL EXAMINATIONS

As soon as you suspect that you're pregnant, notify your doctor and schedule an appointment. This first prenatal examination is typically a long one, and it's a good idea to bring your partner along. The laboratory tests that will be performed and the personal information you provide during the first visit will establish your personal database for your entire pregnancy.

Subsequent visits, which are much shorter, generally involve listening to the unborn baby's heart rate; estimating the baby's size and position; measuring the growth of the uterus; monitoring your blood pressure and weight gain; testing your urine; asking about any symptoms; and answering any questions or concerns you and your partner may have. At specific weeks during your pregnancy, you will also receive additional tests or evaluations. Pregnant women are typically seen by their obstetricians about once a month until the twenty-eighth week, then every other week until the thirty-sixth week, then every week until delivery (usually thirty-nine to forty-one weeks).

Your Baby's Growth

The purpose of prenatal care is to monitor your health and the health of your unborn baby and to detect and treat any problems as soon as possible. Central to both prenatal care and metabolic programming is the goal of optimal fetal growth. Monitoring fetal growth has been made much easier by the use of ultrasound.

ULTRASOUND EXAMINATIONS

One of the wonders of modern medicine, ultrasound allows your doctor to examine your unborn baby safely without disturbing the pregnancy. This technology uses sound waves to create a picture of the fetus, the surrounding fluid, and the placenta. It is performed either by inserting a lubricated probe into the vagina, or by moving a lubricated transducer back and forth across the abdomen. The probe or transducer records the echoes of sound waves bouncing off the baby and the placenta, and displays them on a video screen. Most couples are thrilled to have this early glimpse of their baby, saying that the experience enhances the parent-infant bond and helps to make up for the common aches and pains of pregnancy.

The first ultrasound examination is usually performed at around eighteen to twenty weeks' gestation. It may be done earlier when twins or supertwins are suspected, or when the mother has had vaginal bleeding and the doctor wants to evaluate the status of the pregnancy. Thereafter, ultrasounds may be repeated every month or so, depending on individual circumstances.

One advantage to ultrasound is that it can help to date your pregnancy more accurately. Many women do not know exactly when they conceived, so by measuring the unborn baby's size and comparing it to normal rates of fetal growth, your obstetrician can determine with greater accuracy when the pregnancy began and when your baby is likely to be born—your due date, also called the estimated date of delivery (EDD) or estimated date of confinement (EDC). Ultrasound is also useful for assessing the location and development of the placenta, checking the volume of amniotic fluid, and evaluating any suspected congenital abnormalities. And it greatly reduces the risk of procedures such as amniocentesis and chorionic villus sampling by providing an "inside view" of the fetus's exact position in the womb.

A very thorough examination called the structural ultrasound is usually done at about eighteen to twenty weeks' gestation. This involves a detailed evaluation of the baby's internal and external organs. At this stage of pregnancy your unborn baby is nearly transparent, so it is possible to look at the brain, heart, and spinal cord to determine if they are well formed and growing properly. The structure of the placenta is also examined.

Subsequent ultrasound evaluations are done to monitor your baby's growth, as compared to the baseline data established at the structural ultrasound. The ultrasonographer or radiologist looks at the placenta, gauges the amount of amniotic fluid surrounding the baby, may measure the length and width of your cervix (using either a vaginal probe or an abdominal scan), and evaluates any fetal organ or tissue that was not clearly visible during the structural survey.

The following fetal measurements are also taken:

- *Biparietal diameter:* the distance from temple to temple on your baby's face
- *Head circumference:* the distance around your baby's head at the temples

- *Abdominal circumference:* the distance around your baby's mid-riff at the umbilicus
- *Femur length:* the length of your baby's thighbone from hip to knee

Each of these measurements is compared to a specific norm or standard for each sex, dated in terms of weeks' gestation, and compared to the measurements made during previous ultrasounds. These measurements are then put into one of several equations in order to calculate an estimated fetal weight.

WHY FETAL MEASUREMENTS MATTER

Understand that all parts of your baby do not grow at the same rate. For instance:

- By the end of the first trimester, your baby's head makes up nearly half of his or her body length, and it has achieved about 30 percent of the size it will be by the time your baby is full term. By twenty weeks, the halfway mark, your baby's head will have reached about half its ultimate birth size, and by twenty-eight weeks, the beginning of the third trimester, it will be about three-quarters the size it will be at birth.
- The growth of your baby's abdomen and femurs are slower than that of your baby's head. By the end of the first trimester, your baby's abdominal circumference has reached only about 25 percent and the femur length is only about 20 percent of the size it will be by full term. By twenty weeks, both of these measures will be about 45 percent of their final size, and by twenty-eight weeks, they will be about 70 percent of the size they will be at birth.
- Your unborn baby's growth in weight, by contrast, follows a very different pattern. By the end of the first trimester, your baby's weight is only about 3 percent of what it will be at full term; by twenty weeks, it's only 9 percent of the final birthweight.

By twenty-eight weeks, the beginning of the third trimester, and nearly three-quarters of the way to the full term forty weeks, your baby's weight is only one-third of his or her ultimate birthweight.

To help you follow how well your baby is growing, the tenth, fiftieth, and ninetieth percentiles of growth for head circumference, abdominal circumference, femur length, and fetal weight are shown in Table 4-1.

Head Circumference

The growth of the head represents growth of the brain. Before birth, the head circumference grows at a rate of about 9 millimeters (0.35 inches) per week—a little faster during the first half of pregnancy and a little slower during the second half. Growth of the head and nervous system takes precedence over other parts of the body. So if fetal growth rate slows down during the second half of pregnancy, often the growth of the head is spared at the expense of the abdomen and femur. The result is an infant with a normal-size head but a shorter length, a growth pattern known as asymmetrical growth restriction. When fetal growth has slowed starting from the first trimester or early second trimester, even the head is not spared, resulting in symmetrical growth restriction.

Abdominal Circumference

The abdominal circumference is the factor most closely related to fetal weight. Before birth, the abdominal circumference grows at a rate of about 10 mm (0.40 inches) per week—slower in the first half of pregnancy and faster during the second half. Abdominal circumference includes fetal fat stores and the glycogen (carbohydrate) stores in the liver, both of which are affected quickly and early on in cases of growth restriction. When fetal growth slows down during the third trimester, it can affect the size of the liver, because it is growing most rapidly during this stage of gestation.

Femur Length

Growth of the femur provides a good barometer of long-term growth. Before birth, the femur length increases at a rate of about 2 mm (0.08 inches) per week—slower during the first half and faster during the second half of pregnancy.

As I mentioned earlier, when you have an ultrasound examination, the ultrasonographer or radiologist takes careful measurements of your baby's biparietal diameter and head circumference, abdominal circumference, and femur length, and puts these measurements into an equation to estimate your baby's weight. The answers yield important information about your baby's development.

Femur Length/Abdominal Circumference

One equation uses the abdominal circumference and femur length. The estimated weights based on these two measures are given in Table 4-2. To use this table, locate the femur measurement on the left-hand column and the abdominal circumference across the top, and follow them across and down. Where they intersect is the estimated fetal weight.

Keep in mind that Table 4-2 provides only an estimate of your unborn baby's weight. You are taking a two-dimensional picture and making a three-dimensional estimate from it, so errors in measurement are therefore cubed. As a result, the actual fetal weight may be as much as 20 percent larger or smaller than the estimated weight, with such errors increasing as the pregnancy progresses.

Femur Length/Abdominal Circumference Ratio

After twenty-one weeks' gestation, among babies who have a normal pattern of growth, the femur length and abdominal

TABLE 4-1. IN UTERO FETAL MEASUREMENTS (10TH, 50TH, AND 90TH PERCENTILES)

Weeks' Gestation	HEAD CIRCUMFERENCE (MM)			ABDOMINAL CIRCUMFERENCE (MM)			FEMUR LENGTH (MM)			FETAL WEIGHT (GM)		
	10th %ile	50th %ile	90th %ile	10th %ile	50th %ile	90th %ile	10th %ile	50th %ile	90th %ile	10th %ile	50th %ile	90th %ile
12	72.4	79.4	86.4	57.9	64.1	70.3	8.3	9.5	10.7	48	58	68
13	84.2	91.8	99.4	67.1	75.3	83.5	10.0	11.9	13.8	61	72	85
14	101.0	108.4	115.8	79.7	87.8	95.9	13.4	15.4	17.4	77	93	109
15	105.8	115.1	124.4	90.9	99.5	108.1	15.8	18.2	20.6	97	117	137
16	120.9	128.1	135.3	106.3	114.5	122.7	19.1	21.5	23.9	121	146	171
17	133.8	143.9	154.0	111.9	123.5	135.1	22.5	24.7	26.9	150	181	212
18	145.6	154.4	163.2	124.1	133.4	142.7	25.4	28.0	30.6	185	223	261
19	159.8	166.6	173.4	140.6	147.0	153.4	28.3	30.5	32.7	227	273	319
20	174.6	181.9	189.2	148.5	158.5	168.5	31.4	33.6	35.8	275	331	387
21	183.4	191.8	200.2	156.9	166.9	176.9	33.9	36.3	38.7	331	399	467
22	192.9	201.7	210.5	165.0	175.7	186.4	35.5	38.2	40.9	398	478	559
23	206.9	217.4	227.9	182.4	189.9	197.4	39.4	41.9	44.4	471	568	665
24	218.2	227.9	237.6	185.7	200.9	216.1	41.6	45.0	48.4	556	670	784
25	227.1	234.8	242.5	198.1	205.7	213.3	43.2	45.9	48.6	652	785	918
26	241.6	251.3	261.0	214.3	223.1	231.9	46.4	48.8	51.2	758	913	1,068

Week												
27	252.6	262.7	272.8	218.8	232.5	246.2	48.0	51.3	54.6	875	1,055	1,234
28	274.1	275.0	284.0	230.9	245.7	260.5	50.5	53.2	55.9	1,004	1,210	1,416
29	276.9	284.6	292.3	242.6	252.3	262.0	53.3	56.0	58.7	1,145	1,379	1,613
30	279.9	288.4	296.9	242.3	256.1	269.9	54.0	56.5	59.0	1,294	1,559	1,824
31	291.4	301.0	310.6	261.5	278.1	294.6	58.0	61.1	64.2	1,453	1,751	2,049
32	296.1	307.7	319.3	269.6	282.9	296.2	59.2	61.8	64.4	1,621	1,953	2,285
33	299.9	312.7	325.5	276.6	299.1	321.6	60.5	63.4	66.3	1,794	2,162	2,530
34	305.8	317.1	328.4	289.5	301.6	313.7	61.1	64.2	67.3	1,973	2,377	2,781
35	314.7	326.4	338.1	296.8	314.6	332.4	64.9	67.3	69.7	2,154	2,595	3,036
36	321.8	332.4	343.0	303.2	321.5	339.8	65.7	68.7	71.7	2,335	2,813	3,291
37	320.7	337.4	354.1	308.3	331.2	354.1	67.7	70.4	73.1	2,513	3,028	3,543
38	322.4	337.4	352.3	318.9	336.2	353.5	67.9	71.5	75.1	2,686	3,236	3,786
39	328.0	346.4	364.8	322.6	350.1	377.6	69.0	72.9	76.8	2,851	3,435	4,019
40	337.5	354.1	370.7	346.7	365.9	385.1	72.0	75.1	78.2	3,004	3,619	4,234

Adapted from F. P. Hadlock, R. B. Harrist, J. Martinez-Poyer. (1991). In utero analysis of fetal growth: A sonographic weight standard. *Radiology* 181:129–133. Used with permission. And F. A. Chervenak, G. C. Isaacson, S. Campbell. *Ultrasound in Obstetrics and Gynecology,* vol. 2; pp. 1777–1782.

TABLE 4-2. ESTIMATES OF FETAL WEIGHT (IN GRAMS) BASED ON ABDOMINAL CIRCUMFERENCE AND FEMUR LENGTH

ABDOMINAL CIRCUMFERENCE (CM)

Femur Length (cm)	20.0	20.5	21.0	21.5	22.0	22.5	23.0	23.5	24.0	24.5	25.0	25.5	26.0	26.5	27.0	27.5	28.0	28.5	29.0	29.5	30.0
4.0	663	691	720	751	783	816	851	887	925	964	1006	1048	1093	1139	1188	1239	1291	1346	1403	1463	1525
4.1	680	709	738	769	802	836	871	907	946	986	1027	1070	1115	1162	1211	1262	1315	1371	1429	1489	1551
4.2	697	726	757	788	821	855	891	928	967	1007	1049	1093	1138	1186	1235	1287	1340	1396	1454	1515	1578
4.3	715	745	776	808	841	875	912	949	988	1029	1071	1116	1162	1209	1259	1311	1365	1422	1480	1541	1605
4.4	734	764	795	827	861	896	933	971	1010	1051	1094	1139	1185	1234	1284	1336	1391	1448	1507	1568	1632
4.5	753	783	815	847	882	917	954	993	1033	1074	1118	1163	1210	1259	1309	1362	1417	1474	1534	1596	1660
4.6	772	803	835	868	903	939	976	1015	1056	1098	1142	1187	1235	1284	1335	1388	1444	1501	1561	1623	1688
4.7	792	823	856	889	924	961	999	1038	1079	1122	1166	1212	1260	1310	1361	1415	1471	1529	1589	1652	1717
4.8	812	844	877	911	947	984	1022	1062	1103	1146	1191	1237	1286	1336	1388	1442	1498	1557	1618	1681	1746
4.9	833	865	899	933	969	1007	1046	1086	1128	1171	1216	1263	1312	1363	1415	1470	1527	1585	1647	1710	1776
5.0	855	887	921	956	993	1031	1070	1111	1153	1197	1243	1290	1339	1390	1443	1498	1555	1615	1676	1740	1806
5.1	877	910	944	980	1016	1055	1095	1136	1179	1223	1269	1317	1367	1418	1471	1527	1584	1644	1706	1770	1837
5.2	899	933	967	1004	1041	1080	1120	1162	1205	1250	1296	1344	1395	1447	1500	1556	1614	1674	1737	1801	1868
5.3	922	956	992	1028	1066	1105	1146	1188	1232	1277	1324	1373	1423	1476	1530	1586	1645	1705	1768	1833	1900
5.4	946	981	1016	1053	1091	1131	1172	1215	1259	1305	1352	1401	1452	1505	1560	1617	1675	1736	1799	1865	1933
5.5	971	1005	1041	1079	1118	1158	1199	1242	1287	1333	1381	1431	1482	1535	1591	1648	1707	1768	1832	1897	1966
5.6	995	1031	1067	1105	1144	1185	1227	1271	1316	1362	1411	1461	1513	1566	1622	1679	1739	1801	1864	1931	1999
5.7	1021	1057	1094	1132	1172	1213	1255	1299	1345	1392	1441	1491	1544	1598	1654	1712	1772	1834	1898	1964	2033
5.8	1047	1084	1121	1160	1200	1242	1285	1329	1375	1422	1472	1523	1575	1630	1686	1744	1805	1867	1932	1999	2068
5.9	1074	1111	1149	1188	1229	1271	1314	1359	1406	1454	1503	1555	1608	1663	1719	1778	1839	1902	1966	2034	2103
6.0	1102	1139	1178	1217	1258	1301	1345	1390	1437	1485	1535	1587	1641	1696	1753	1812	1873	1936	2002	2069	2139
6.1	1130	1168	1207	1247	1289	1331	1376	1421	1469	1518	1568	1620	1674	1730	1788	1847	1908	1972	2038	2105	2175
6.2	1160	1198	1237	1278	1319	1363	1408	1454	1501	1551	1602	1654	1709	1765	1823	1882	1944	2008	2074	2142	2212
6.3	1189	1228	1268	1309	1351	1395	1440	1487	1535	1585	1636	1689	1744	1800	1858	1919	1981	2045	2111	2180	2250
6.4	1220	1259	1299	1341	1384	1428	1473	1520	1569	1619	1671	1724	1779	1836	1895	1956	2018	2082	2149	2218	2289
6.5	1251	1291	1332	1373	1417	1461	1507	1555	1604	1655	1707	1760	1816	1873	1932	1993	2056	2121	2188	2256	2328
6.6	1284	1324	1365	1407	1451	1496	1542	1590	1640	1691	1743	1797	1853	1911	1970	2031	2094	2160	2227	2296	2367
6.7	1317	1357	1399	1441	1486	1531	1578	1626	1676	1728	1780	1835	1891	1949	2009	2070	2134	2199	2267	2336	2408
6.8	1351	1391	1433	1477	1521	1567	1615	1663	1713	1765	1819	1873	1930	1988	2048	2110	2174	2240	2307	2377	2449
6.9	1385	1427	1469	1513	1558	1604	1652	1701	1752	1804	1857	1913	1970	2028	2089	2151	2215	2281	2348	2418	2490
7.0	1421	1463	1506	1550	1595	1642	1690	1740	1791	1843	1897	1953	2010	2069	2130	2192	2256	2322	2391	2461	2533
7.1	1458	1500	1543	1588	1633	1681	1729	1779	1830	1883	1938	1994	2051	2110	2171	2234	2299	2365	2433	2504	2576
7.2	1495	1538	1581	1626	1672	1720	1769	1819	1871	1924	1979	2035	2093	2153	2214	2277	2342	2408	2477	2547	2620
7.3	1534	1577	1621	1666	1713	1761	1810	1861	1913	1966	2021	2078	2136	2196	2258	2321	2386	2453	2521	2592	2665
7.4	1573	1616	1661	1707	1754	1802	1852	1903	1955	2009	2065	2122	2180	2240	2302	2365	2431	2498	2566	2637	2710
7.5	1614	1657	1699	1745	1791	1845	1895	1946	1999	2053	2109	2166	2225	2285	2347	2411	2476	2543	2612	2683	2756
7.6	1655	1699	1742	1788	1835	1888	1939	1990	2043	2098	2154	2211	2270	2331	2393	2457	2523	2590	2659	2730	2803
7.7	1698	1742	1786	1835	1883	1933	1983	2035	2089	2144	2200	2258	2317	2378	2440	2504	2570	2638	2707	2778	2851
7.8	1741	1786	1833	1880	1928	1978	2029	2082	2135	2191	2247	2305	2365	2426	2488	2553	2618	2686	2755	2827	2899
7.9	1786	1832	1878	1926	1975	2025	2076	2129	2183	2238	2295	2353	2413	2474	2537	2602	2668	2735	2805	2876	2949
8.0	1832	1878	1925	1973	2022	2073	2124	2177	2232	2287	2344	2403	2463	2524	2587	2652	2718	2785	2855	2926	2999
8.1	1879	1926	1973	2021	2071	2121	2173	2227	2282	2337	2394	2453	2513	2575	2638	2702	2769	2837	2906	2977	3050
8.2	1928	1974	2022	2071	2120	2171	2224	2277	2332	2388	2446	2504	2565	2626	2690	2754	2821	2889	2958	3029	3102
8.3	1978	2024	2072	2121	2171	2223	2275	2329	2384	2440	2498	2557	2617	2679	2743	2807	2874	2942	3011	3082	3155

ABDOMINAL CIRCUMFERENCE (CM)

Femur Length (cm)	30.5	31.0	31.5	32.0	32.5	33.0	33.5	34.0	34.5	35.0	35.5	36.0	36.5	37.0	37.5	38.0	38.5	39.0	39.5	40.0
4.0	1590	1658	1729	1802	1879	1959	2042	2129	2220	2314	2413	2515	2622	2734	2850	2972	3098	3230	3367	3511
4.1	1617	1685	1756	1830	1907	1987	2071	2158	2249	2344	2442	2545	2652	2764	2880	3002	3128	3260	3397	3540
4.2	1644	1712	1783	1858	1935	2016	2100	2187	2279	2373	2472	2575	2683	2794	2911	3032	3159	3290	3427	3570
4.3	1671	1740	1812	1886	1964	2045	2129	2217	2308	2404	2503	2606	2713	2825	2942	3063	3189	3321	3458	3600
4.4	1699	1768	1840	1915	1993	2075	2159	2247	2339	2434	2533	2637	2744	2856	2973	3094	3220	3352	3488	3630
4.5	1727	1797	1869	1944	2023	2105	2189	2278	2370	2465	2565	2668	2776	2888	3004	3125	3251	3383	3519	3661
4.6	1756	1826	1898	1974	2053	2135	2220	2309	2401	2497	2595	2700	2807	2919	3036	3157	3283	3414	3550	3692
4.7	1785	1855	1928	2004	2084	2166	2251	2340	2432	2528	2623	2720	2840	2952	3068	3189	3315	3446	3582	3723
4.8	1814	1885	1959	2035	2115	2197	2283	2372	2464	2560	2660	2764	2872	2984	3100	3221	3347	3478	3613	3754
4.9	1845	1916	1990	2066	2146	2229	2315	2404	2497	2593	2693	2797	2905	3017	3133	3254	3380	3510	3645	3786
5.0	1875	1947	2021	2098	2178	2261	2347	2437	2530	2626	2725	2830	2938	3050	3166	3287	3412	3542	3677	3818
5.1	1906	1978	2053	2130	2210	2294	2380	2470	2563	2659	2760	2864	2972	3084	3200	3320	3445	3575	3710	3850
5.2	1938	2010	2085	2163	2243	2327	2413	2503	2597	2693	2794	2898	3006	3117	3234	3354	3479	3608	3743	3882
5.3	1970	2043	2118	2196	2277	2360	2447	2537	2631	2728	2823	2922	3040	3152	3268	3388	3513	3642	3776	3915
5.4	2003	2076	2151	2229	2311	2395	2482	2572	2665	2762	2863	2967	3075	3186	3302	3422	3547	3676	3809	3948
5.5	2036	2109	2185	2264	2345	2429	2516	2607	2700	2797	2898	3002	3110	3221	3337	3457	3581	3710	3843	3981
5.6	2070	2143	2220	2298	2380	2464	2552	2642	2736	2833	2933	3038	3145	3257	3372	3492	3616	3744	3877	4015
5.7	2104	2178	2254	2333	2415	2500	2587	2678	2772	2869	2970	3074	3181	3293	3408	3527	3651	3779	3911	4048
5.8	2139	2213	2290	2369	2451	2536	2624	2714	2808	2905	3006	3110	3218	3329	3444	3563	3686	3814	3946	4082
5.9	2175	2249	2326	2405	2488	2573	2660	2751	2845	2942	3043	3147	3254	3366	3480	3599	3722	3849	3981	4117
6.0	2211	2286	2363	2442	2525	2610	2698	2789	2883	2980	3080	3184	3292	3403	3517	3636	3758	3885	4016	4151
6.1	2248	2323	2400	2480	2562	2647	2736	2827	2921	3018	3118	3222	3329	3440	3554	3673	3795	3921	4052	4186
6.2	2285	2360	2438	2518	2600	2686	2774	2865	2959	3056	3157	3260	3367	3478	3592	3710	3832	3957	4087	4222
6.3	2323	2398	2476	2556	2639	2725	2813	2904	2998	3095	3195	3299	3405	3516	3630	3747	3869	3994	4124	4257
6.4	2362	2437	2515	2595	2678	2764	2852	2943	3037	3134	3235	3338	3445	3555	3668	3785	3906	4031	4160	4293
6.5	2401	2477	2555	2635	2718	2804	2892	2983	3077	3174	3274	3378	3484	3594	3707	3824	3944	4069	4197	4329
6.6	2441	2517	2595	2675	2759	2844	2932	3024	3118	3215	3315	3418	3524	3633	3746	3863	3981	4106	4234	4366
6.7	2481	2557	2636	2716	2800	2885	2974	3065	3159	3256	3355	3458	3564	3673	3786	3902	4031	4144	4271	4402
6.8	2523	2599	2677	2758	2841	2927	3016	3107	3201	3297	3397	3499	3605	3714	3826	3941	4069	4183	4309	4439
6.9	2564	2641	2719	2800	2884	2969	3058	3149	3242	3339	3438	3541	3646	3754	3866	3981	4106	4222	4347	4477
7.0	2607	2683	2762	2843	2927	3012	3101	3192	3285	3381	3481	3583	3688	3796	3907	4022	4144	4261	4386	4514
7.1	2650	2727	2806	2887	2969	3056	3144	3235	3328	3424	3523	3625	3730	3838	3948	4062	4183	4300	4425	4552
7.2	2694	2771	2850	2931	3014	3100	3188	3279	3372	3468	3567	3668	3772	3880	3990	4104	4222	4340	4464	4591
7.3	2739	2816	2895	2976	3059	3145	3233	3323	3416	3512	3610	3712	3816	3922	4032	4145	4261	4381	4503	4629
7.4	2785	2861	2940	3021	3105	3190	3278	3369	3461	3557	3655	3755	3859	3966	4075	4187	4300	4421	4543	4668
7.5	2831	2908	2987	3068	3151	3236	3324	3414	3507	3602	3700	3800	3903	4009	4118	4230	4340	4462	4583	4708
7.6	2878	2955	3034	3115	3198	3283	3371	3461	3553	3648	3745	3845	3948	4053	4161	4272	4381	4504	4624	4747
7.7	2926	3003	3081	3162	3245	3331	3418	3508	3600	3694	3791	3891	3993	4098	4205	4316	4421	4545	4665	4787
7.8	2974	3051	3130	3211	3294	3379	3466	3555	3647	3741	3838	3937	4039	4143	4250	4360	4462	4588	4706	4827
7.9	3024	3100	3179	3260	3343	3427	3514	3604	3695	3789	3885	3984	4085	4188	4295	4404	4504	4630	4748	4868
8.0	3074	3151	3229	3310	3392	3477	3564	3653	3744	3837	3933	4031	4131	4234	4340	4448	4545	4673	4790	4909
8.1	3125	3202	3280	3360	3443	3527	3614	3702	3793	3886	3981	4079	4179	4281	4386	4493	4588	4716	4832	4950
8.2	3177	3253	3332	3412	3494	3578	3664	3752	3843	3935	4030	4127	4226	4328	4432	4539	4630	4760	4875	4992
8.3	3230	3306	3384	3464	3546	3630	3716	3803	3893	3985	4080	4175	4275	4376	4479	4585	4716	4804	4918	5034

Adapted from F. P. Hadlock, R. B. Harrist, R. J. Carpenter, et al. (1984). Sonographic estimation of fetal weight. *Radiology*; 150:535–540. Used with permission circumference remain in fairly constant proportion to each other, regardless of gestational age. Expressed as femur length (in centimeters) divided by abdominal circumference (in centimeters) times 100, ratios above the range of 20 to 24 indicate intrauterine growth restriction[2]. This type of slowed growth is associated with an increased risk for preterm labor and delivery, particularly for babies who are symmetrically small. Among pregnancies complicated by preterm labor treated with tocolytics (medications to stop labor), the babies who were ultimately born at full term had significantly lower (more normal) femur length/abdominal circumference ratios. Those babies who were delivered preterm had higher (less normal) ratios[3]. This means that preterm labor that does not respond to tocolytic therapy is associated with impaired fetal growth[4]. In other words, when an unborn baby has this type of growth restriction, and labor begins prematurely, efforts to halt labor with medication are less likely to succeed.

Head Circumference/Abdominal Circumference Ratio

Another ratio that can indicate when growth is not proceeding normally is the head circumference to abdominal circumference ratio[5]. If the head is growing at a normal rate and abdominal circumference rate is slowing down, the ratio will be higher than normal. This occurs with asymmetrical growth restriction. With slowed growth of both body parts, the ratio will be lower than normal. This indicates symmetrical growth restriction, which occurs when growth is slowed from early in pregnancy until delivery.

METABOLIC PROGRAMMING AND FETAL GROWTH

When the baby is growing at a normal rate, when head and abdominal circumference and femur length all consistently match gestational age, when the mother's health is good, and when she is gaining weight at an appropriate rate, the baby's risk of poor health at birth or beyond is greatly reduced. But when fetal growth slows down, for any of a number of reasons, the risk to the baby is significantly increased both in infancy and later in life. The specific risks depend on the stage of pregnancy at which the baby's growth rate has slowed.

First Trimester: Conception to Twelve Weeks

When growth slows down early in pregnancy due to a chromosomal abnormality, infection, low maternal prepregnancy weight, or low weight gain, the baby adapts by slowing down its overall growth. All measurements, including head circumference, are less than normal for the stage of pregnancy, a condition termed small for gestational age, or SGA. This type of growth is associated with a higher risk of preterm labor and preterm birth.

At birth, the baby's weight and all body proportions are reduced, resulting in a symmetrically small baby. During infancy, growth will continue to be slow, with weight and size still lagging behind by one year of age. In the context of long-term metabolic programming, this type of fetal growth is associated with an increased risk for hypertension during adulthood.

Second Trimester: Thirteen to Twenty-seven Weeks

Sometimes fetal growth proceeds normally during the first trimester but then slows down in the second trimester. This can happen when the mother overexerts herself physically, suffers from work-related fatigue, gains too little weight, develops iron-deficiency anemia, or contracts an infection. The baby adapts by developing insulin resistance; the cells of his body become less sensitive to the action of insulin. This type of growth is also associated with an increased risk for preterm birth[6,7,8].

As a result, the baby's weight at birth is reduced, but body length and head circumference are normal. These characteristics exemplify a thin baby. During infancy, the thin baby's growth will catch up so that by one year of age the child's weight should be normal. However, he or she will remain at increased risk for hypertension, non-insulin-dependent diabetes, and cardiovascular disease during adult life.

Third Trimester: Twenty-eight to Forty Weeks

When growth begins to slow down during the third trimester, the reasons are often similar to those described for the second trimester: excessive physical activity by the mother, low weight gain, fatigue, or iron-deficiency anemia. When this occurs, the unborn baby adapts by sustaining brain growth at the expense of the rest of the body. The thymus, which is vital to regulating the body's immune response, is one of the organs that may suffer with this pattern of altered growth[9,10].

This type of baby has a normal birthweight, but is short, or stunted, for gestational age. In infancy, his or her growth will continue to lag behind. During childhood, he or she will be at increased risk for developing asthma[11], and will also be more susceptible to infection. As an adult, he or she will have an elevated risk for many serious health problems, including hypertension, non-insulin-dependent diabetes, high cholesterol, and cardiovascular disease.

Prenatal Tests

Fortunately, there's a great deal you can do to lower your unborn baby's future health risks. One vital step toward positive programming is to comply with your obstetrician's instructions, including whatever prenatal tests he or she may recommend. You may want to use Table 4-3 to keep track of the laboratory and diagnostic tests you undergo, filling in the test dates and results as your pregnancy progresses.

TABLE 4-3. PRENATAL SCHEDULE OF EXAMINATIONS AND TESTS

Initial Labs	Date	Result
Blood Type		
Rh Type		
Antibody Screen		
Hemoglobin/Hematocrit		
Pap Smear		
Rubella		
Syphilis		
Gonnorhoa		
Urine Culture/Screen		
HBsAG		

8 to 18 Weeks Labs	Date	Result
Ultrasound		
MSAFP		
Amniocentesis/CVS		
Karyotype		
Alpha-Fetoprotein		

24 to 28 Weeks Labs	Date	Result
Hemoglobin/Hematocrit		
Diabetes Screen		
Glucose Tolerance Test		
Rh Antibody Screen		

Rhogam (at 28 weeks)

32 to 36 Weeks Labs	Date	Result
Ultrasound		
Syphilis		
Gonnorhea		
Hemoglobin/Hematocrit		

Optional Labs	Date	Result
HIV		
Hemoglobin Electrophoresis		
Chlamydia		
Other		

WHAT TO EXPECT FROM PRENATAL TESTS

Today's medical testing technologies are a boon to your unborn baby's metabolic programming. They provide important information to help assure the baby's proper development, as well as to safeguard your own health. Here's what to expect.

Pelvic Examination

During your first prenatal visit, your obstetrician will perform a pelvic examination to estimate how many weeks pregnant you are and to detect any problems. He or she will also take a Pap smear, which entails scraping a few cells from your cervix to be examined under a microscope for any abnormal cervical changes. Generally, a pelvic examination is part of the initial prenatal visit and is not done again until after twenty-four weeks' gestation, unless you develop a vaginal infection or experience symptoms of preterm labor such as uterine contractions or pelvic pressure.

Blood Tests

Blood will be drawn to evaluate your hemoglobin and hematocrit (a check for anemia). If you are anemic, you can increase your iron through changes in your diet. Remember, as discussed in Chapter 2, you should eat six servings of iron-rich protein foods (beef, lamb, pork) and eight servings of iron-rich breads and grains each day.

You'll also be evaluated for Rh factor. If your blood is Rh negative and your partner's is Rh positive, this can potentially cause problems for your unborn baby, particularly if this is not your first pregnancy. To prevent you from making antibodies against your unborn baby, your doctor may give you injections of a drug called Rho (D) Immuno Globulin (Human), or Rhogam, at about twenty-eight weeks' gestation and/or immediately after delivery.

Blood tests can also detect the presence of hepatitis B, syphilis, gonorrhea, and HIV antibodies. Since these infections can be passed on to your unborn baby and cause serious harm, it's important that they be diagnosed and treated. These blood tests may be repeated later in pregnancy if necessary.

You will also be tested for gestational diabetes between weeks twenty-six and twenty eight. This test involves drinking a special high-carbohydrate beverage and having a sample of your blood drawn one hour later. If your blood glucose level is high during this screening test, you will be scheduled to take an oral glucose tolerance test (OGTT). To prepare, you fast overnight. Then your blood is drawn. Next, you drink the high-carbohydrate beverage. More blood is drawn after one hour, two hours, and three hours. If the results indicate high levels of blood glucose in two or more of these blood samples, you may be given a special diet or even placed on insulin until the end of your pregnancy.

This may seem like a lot of tests, but in fact your blood will probably be drawn only a few times during your pregnancy. One sample of blood can often be used for more than one test. And of course, the information these tests provide is very important to your baby's well-being.

Urine Tests

At each prenatal visit your urine will be tested for the presence of ketones and protein and, if you are experiencing pain on urination or other urinary symptoms, for white blood cells. The purpose is to check for signs of pregnancy-induced hypertension or infection. The presence of ketones in the urine also indicates that you may not be getting enough calories in your diet and that you need to eat more or more often.

Amniocentesis

This procedure has been used for more than thirty years. It is now routinely recommended for women age 35 and older, when the risks of age-related pregnancy problems increase significantly. Amniocentesis is also recommended when there is a family history of chromosomal abnormalities or neural tube defects, or when the mother has a history of miscarriage.

Before birth your baby is floating in a liquid called amniotic fluid. As the fetus grows, cells from its body are discarded into the amniotic fluid. During amniocentesis, fluid containing these discarded cells is retrieved so that the genetic material they contain can be evaluated. Amniocentesis is generally performed between the fourteenth and twentieth weeks of gestation. Before fourteen weeks there is not enough amniotic fluid. After twenty weeks, it is much more difficult to perform a therapeutic abortion in the event a couple decides to end the pregnancy based on the test results. This procedure also may be done in the case of premature labor in order to determine if the baby's lungs are mature enough to breathe. This test is also used to evaluate a medical problem that requires the baby to be delivered early.

Using ultrasound, the fetus's image is projected on a screen.

After cleaning your skin with an antiseptic, the obstetrician inserts a long, very thin needle through your abdomen and into your uterus, and withdraws some of the amniotic fluid from the baby's amniotic sac. (Most women experience only slight cramping, though the procedure does carry a small risk of infection, premature labor, or even loss of the pregnancy.) The amniotic fluid is sent to a special laboratory where the cells are cultured and then examined for chromosomal abnormalities. Test results are usually available within two weeks. The test also reveals your baby's sex, so you can opt to have that information before the birth if you'd like.

Chorionic Villus Sampling

Chorionic villi are part of the chorion, which eventually becomes the part of the placenta closest to the baby. Because the chorionic villus contains the baby's genetic material, it can be tested for a wide variety of congenital conditions. Chorionic villus sampling is done as early as the eighth week of pregnancy and up to the twelfth week, and the results of the test are usually available within two weeks. This is an advantage over amniocentesis because, if results are abnormal, the pregnancy can be terminated during the first trimester when therapeutic abortion is most safe. Also, the relatively early diagnosis allows a couple to make this difficult decision more privately, before family and friends may even be aware of the pregnancy.

The procedure for chorionic villus sampling is similar to that of amniocentesis. Guided by ultrasound, the doctor inserts a long, thin needle either through your abdomen, or through the vagina and cervix, to obtain a sample of the chorionic villi. After the procedure, a woman may experience slight bleeding, which is not cause for concern unless it lasts longer than two days. The risk of miscarriage is about the same as with amniocentesis.

Alpha-fetoprotein Test
Alpha-fetoprotein is a type of protein produced only by an unborn baby or its yolk sac. The test, which is performed at sixteen to eighteen weeks' gestation, involves analyzing the level of this protein in the mother's blood. High levels suggest that the pregnancy is farther along than previously estimated; that there is more than one fetus; or that the baby may have a neural tube defect. Low levels of alpha-fetoprotein indicate an increased possibility of Down's syndrome or other chromosomal problem. Unlike amniocentesis and chorionic villus sampling, alpha-fetoprotein is only a screening test, not a diagnostic procedure. Abnormal results indicate that further testing should be done.

Non-stress Tests
Non-stress tests may or may not be utilized, depending on the circumstances of the individual pregnancy. The purpose of this test is to evaluate the unborn baby's heartbeat and movements and the frequency of uterine contractions using external fetal monitors. If the baby's heart rate does not react to movement, or if the baby does not move at all, or if other abnormalities are noted, fetal distress may be present. This type of test is typically performed toward the end of pregnancy, although if the estimated weight of your unborn baby is below the tenth percentile, non-stress tests may be ordered earlier and more frequently. There are two common types, the biophysical profile and the Doppler flow studies.

The biophysical profile, which takes about thirty minutes, combines the information from the non-stress test with the results of an ultrasound. The biophysical profile includes an assessment of your unborn baby's heart rate, breathing patterns, body movements, muscle tone, and amount of amniotic fluid. The heart rate is measured using the non-stress test, and ultrasound is used to determine the other measurements. Each of these measurements is given a score and totaled. A score of 8 to 10 is normal; if the score is less than 8, you may need to repeat the test the next day.

Doppler flow studies may be used in cases where a baby's growth has slowed, the heart rate has dropped, the baby's activity has decreased, or the amount of amniotic fluid is unusually low or high. This test uses a form of ultrasound that converts sound waves into signals, in order to evaluate the quality of blood flow through the umbilical cord.

Your Commitment to Prenatal Care

With this knowledge of fetal growth and development, an appreciation for the importance of proper prenatal care, and a commitment to following your doctor's advice, you are boosting your baby's odds of being born healthy and staying healthy for decades.

What you do now—every day, every week, and every month that you are pregnant—influences your child's well-being for a lifetime. The following chapters will guide you through your pregnancy, as well as your baby's childhood and adolescence, so you can take positive steps toward programming your baby for a healthy future.

5 ⚘ THE FIRST TRIMESTER

Pregnancy is divided into three trimesters, time periods of about three months each. The first trimester, also called the embryonic period, includes the time from conception to the twelfth week of pregnancy.

I want to state emphatically that *the first trimester is the most critical time for your baby's metabolic programming because all of the body's essential internal and external structures are beginning to form.* Cells and systems are most susceptible to the effects of metabolic programming when they are growing rapidly, and right now, your baby's cells are not only increasing greatly in number, but they are also differentiating into various cell types. Anything that disrupts normal development at this stage could lead to malformations and birth defects, or even loss of the pregnancy.

For instance, if the baby is undernourished during the time at which fetal cells are differentiating, the result can be a permanent alteration in the structure and function of the organs these cells will go on to form. These adaptations ensure continued survival and growth, but at the expense of longevity—because they set the stage for the subsequent development of chronic disease. The heart, brain, and nervous system are most likely to be adversely affected.

Two Nutrients Your Baby Needs Right Now

The dietary advise outlined in Chapter 2 is particularly important in the first trimester. *During the first three months of pregnancy, 70 percent of the nutrients you supply to your developing baby are devoted to brain growth.* More than half of the brain is composed of fat. Since DHA (an omega-3 essential fatty acid) is the most abundant type of fat present, it is essential that you have adequate amounts of this nutrient in your diet. The best sources of DHA include all types of fish and seafood (see Chapter 2 for more information).

The other key nutrient in programming your baby's neurological health now is folic acid. With some creativity you can easily increase your intake of folic acid–rich foods. Helena, a mother of two, reports, "I wasn't a fruit and veggie eater before I got pregnant, but I found some simple ways to increase my folic acid intake. One favorite strategy was to add tomatoes, cucumbers, and bean sprouts to my sandwiches. Another was to double the beans in my chili recipe. I also learned to love green and red peppers stir-fried with beef."

Remember, too, that the placenta is developing rapidly during this time. The placenta is the vital middleman between you and your child because it delivers nutrients from your bloodstream to your unborn baby and carries away the waste products. Any factors that interfere with placental growth now will adversely affect your baby's growth later in pregnancy. To help the placenta develop properly, be sure to get plenty of protein and foods rich in iron.

The First-Trimester Baby

To fully understand why metabolic programming is so significant in the first trimester, it's helpful to review the basics of how your unborn baby develops, from the moment of conception through the next several months.

CONCEPTION: A QUICK REVIEW

Every month during a woman's childbearing years (from menarche to menopause), her ovaries release a mature egg, or ovum, in a process called ovulation. This egg carries the woman's genetic material, a complement of twenty-three chromosomes, as well as a supply of nutrients. The ovum then begins to travel slowly down one of the Fallopian tubes on its way to the uterus.

The father's complement of twenty-three chromosomes is carried in his sperm. Slender and much smaller than the ovum, each one of millions of sperm tries to make its way from the cervix, up through the uterus, and into the Fallopian tubes. The energy for this trip, which can take from one to six hours, comes from each sperm's sparse nutrient stores. But before a sperm can fertilize the ovum, it must undergo a series of changes, similar to removing a protective coat, which are stimulated mainly by the male hormone testosterone. Small perforations are formed at each sperm's tip to permit the escape of enzymes, which in turn allow the head of the sperm to penetrate the surface of the ovum.

The moment of the sperm's penetration into the ovum is called fertilization or conception. Immediate changes occur within the ovum inhibiting the entry of more sperm. The chromosomes from both mother and father then unite to form a zygote, which is a Greek term meaning "yoked together." The sex of the just-conceived baby has already been determined at this stage. If the ovum was penetrated by a sperm bearing an X chromosome, a girl is formed; if it was penetrated by a sperm bearing a Y chromosome, a boy is formed.

Sometimes a woman's ovaries release two separate eggs at about the same time. If both are fertilized by separate sperm, the result is fraternal (nonidentical) twins. Less frequently, a single egg that has already been fertilized by a single sperm will divide soon after conception, resulting in identical twins.

YOUR BABY'S DUE DATE

With a singleton pregnancy, the date of birth usually occurs about 266 days after conception. That's equal to about 38 weeks, 8¾ calendar months, or 9½ lunar months. But because the exact time of fertilization is often not known (except in the case of infertility treatments), the expected date of delivery is usually calculated from the first day of the last menstrual period (LMP). This is why we speak of pregnancy as lasting approximately 280 days, 40 weeks, 9 calendar months, or 10 lunar months.

If yours is a multiple-gestation pregnancy, you will probably deliver sooner. Twins, on average, are born at thirty-six weeks' gestation. Triplets typically arrive at thirty-two weeks, while quadruplet pregnancies generally last about thirty weeks.

To calculate your due date, check your records for the date of the first day of your last period. Then refer to Table 5-1. Locate your LMP (month and day) in the appropriate row of bold type. Directly below that date is your due date.

WEEK-BY-WEEK GROWTH AND DEVELOPMENT

Here's a description of your unborn baby's fascinating first-trimester development. At no other time during life does the human body grow and change so rapidly—nor offer so many opportunities to maximize the positive effects of metabolic programming.

Week One

Your monthly menstruation takes place. By the end of the week, bleeding has stopped.

TABLE 5-1. CALCULATING YOUR DUE DATE

	1	2	3	4	5	6	7	8	9	10	11	12	13	14	15	16	17	18	19	20	21	22	23	24	25	26	27	28	29	30	31
January	1	2	3	4	5	6	7	8	9	10	11	12	13	14	15	16	17	18	19	20	21	22	23	24	25	26	27	28	29	30	31
October/November	8	9	10	11	12	13	14	15	16	17	18	19	20	21	22	23	24	25	26	27	28	29	30	31	1	2	3	4	5	6	7
February	1	2	3	4	5	6	7	8	9	10	11	12	13	14	15	16	17	18	19	20	21	22	23	24	25	26	27	28			
November/December	8	9	10	11	12	13	14	15	16	17	18	19	20	21	22	23	24	25	26	27	28	29	30	1	2	3	4	5			
March	1	2	3	4	5	6	7	8	9	10	11	12	13	14	15	16	17	18	19	20	21	22	23	24	25	26	27	28	29	30	31
December/January	6	7	8	9	10	11	12	13	14	15	16	17	18	19	20	21	22	23	24	25	26	27	28	29	30	31	1	2	3	4	5
April	1	2	3	4	5	6	7	8	9	10	11	12	13	14	15	16	17	18	19	20	21	22	23	24	25	26	27	28	29	30	
January/February	6	7	8	9	10	11	12	13	14	15	16	17	18	19	20	21	22	23	24	25	26	27	28	29	30	31	1	2	3	4	
May	1	2	3	4	5	6	7	8	9	10	11	12	13	14	15	16	17	18	19	20	21	22	23	24	25	26	27	28	29	30	31
February/March	5	6	7	8	9	10	11	12	13	14	15	16	17	18	19	20	21	22	23	24	25	26	27	28	1	2	3	4	5	6	7
June	1	2	3	4	5	6	7	8	9	10	11	12	13	14	15	16	17	18	19	20	21	22	23	24	25	26	27	28	29	30	
March/April	8	9	10	11	12	13	14	15	16	17	18	19	20	21	22	23	24	25	26	27	28	29	30	31	1	2	3	4	5	6	
July	1	2	3	4	5	6	7	8	9	10	11	12	13	14	15	16	17	18	19	20	21	22	23	24	25	26	27	28	29	30	31
April/May	7	8	9	10	11	12	13	14	15	16	17	18	19	20	21	22	23	24	25	26	27	28	29	30	1	2	3	4	5	6	7
August	1	2	3	4	5	6	7	8	9	10	11	12	13	14	15	16	17	18	19	20	21	22	23	24	25	26	27	28	29	30	31
May/June	8	9	10	11	12	13	14	15	16	17	18	19	20	21	22	23	24	25	26	27	28	29	30	31	1	2	3	4	5	6	7
September	1	2	3	4	5	6	7	8	9	10	11	12	13	14	15	16	17	18	19	20	21	22	23	24	25	26	27	28	29	30	
June/July	8	9	10	11	12	13	14	15	16	17	18	19	20	21	22	23	24	25	26	27	28	29	30	31	1	2	3	4	5	6	
October	1	2	3	4	5	6	7	8	9	10	11	12	13	14	15	16	17	18	19	20	21	22	23	24	25	26	27	28	29	30	31
July/August	8	9	10	11	12	13	14	15	16	17	18	19	20	21	22	23	24	25	26	27	28	29	30	31	1	2	3	4	5	6	7
November	1	2	3	4	5	6	7	8	9	10	11	12	13	14	15	16	17	18	19	20	21	22	23	24	25	26	27	28	29	30	
August/September	8	9	10	11	12	13	14	15	16	17	18	19	20	21	22	23	24	25	26	27	28	29	30	31	1	2	3	4	5	6	
December	1	2	3	4	5	6	7	8	9	10	11	12	13	14	15	16	17	18	19	20	21	22	23	24	25	26	27	28	29	30	31
September/October	7	8	9	10	11	12	13	14	15	16	17	18	19	20	21	22	23	24	25	26	27	28	29	30	1	2	3	4	5	6	7

Week Two

The endometrium, or the lining of the uterus, begins to build up again in preparation for a possible pregnancy. Ovulation occurs, followed by conception. Over the next several days, the zygote makes the four-inch journey down the Fallopian tube, its cells dividing and doubling in number, until it arrives in the uterus. Bathed in fluid from within the uterus, the zygote separates into outer and inner layers. The outer layer will grow to form the major portion of the placenta. The inner layer will grow to become the embryo, the unborn baby.

Week Three

Up to this point, most of the food supply for the developing embryo has come from nutrients stored within the ovum and from the surrounding fluids. By the end of the first week after conception, the developing embryo is delicately implanted in the lining of the uterus and surrounded by tissue rich in carbohydrate, an effect of the hormone progesterone. The fertilized egg typically implants in the upper third of the uterus. With implantation some bleeding may occur, which some new mothers-to-be may mistake as a light period.

The fertilized egg continues to rapidly divide into clusters of several hundreds of cells, each destined for a specific function. The placenta begins producing human chorionic gonadotropin hormone (HCG), which maintains the growth of the endometrium by keeping levels of estrogen and progesterone high. HCG is released into the mother's bloodstream and urine, and by the end of the third week the presence of this hormone can be detected by a pregnancy test.

Week Four

The placenta has grown deeper into the endometrium. As the mother's blood supply bathes the outside of the placenta and the baby's circulation flows within, the placenta passes vital nutrients to your child and carries away waste.

The egg has grown from 0.006 of an inch to 0.3 of an inch, from a single cell to millions of cells. These cells begin to differentiate into three types of tissues: those that will become the nervous system, hair, and skin; those that will become the gastrointestinal tract; and those that will become muscles, bones, and blood vessels.

Week Five
The embryo's heart and circulatory system begin to evolve. Any remaining nutrients from the ovum are quickly being depleted, so the embryo must receive oxygen and nutrients from the mother's circulation. By the end of this week the baby's umbilical cord—the vital link to the placenta—has formed, containing three distinct blood vessels. Once the embryo's blood supply has been established, growth can begin in earnest.

The spinal cord and nervous system are also developing rapidly now. Along the length of the embryo's tiny body, cells stack up to begin to form the spinal cord and backbone.

Week Six
By now the early stages of heart formation are complete and the baby's heart has begun to beat. Soon the embryo will start to produce its own blood. Meanwhile, the limbs are forming. By the twenty-sixth day after conception, the baby has the beginnings of arms. By day twenty-eight, budding legs are visible.

Weeks Seven and Eight
Rapid cellular growth during this time causes a significant event to occur—a "folding" of the developing embryo, which now assumes a more tubular, C-shaped curvature. The eyes develop and become pigmented. The outer ears and fingers start to take shape, and soon after the early beginnings of toes become apparent. The kidneys and gastrointestinal tract are beginning to form. By the

end of the second month, the baby is about one inch in length and weighs about 0.14 ounce (4 grams).

Weeks Nine and Ten

The fingers, toes, and outer ears become more developed. By the close of the tenth week—the end of the embryonic period—all major organs have been formed. A space called the amniotic cavity, which had formed between the embryo and the inner lining of the placenta, has gradually filled with fluid to become the amniotic sac, or bag of waters. The developing embryo floats in this sac as he or she grows, cushioned from shocks from the outside environment and kept at an even temperature.

Weeks Eleven and Twelve

The baby is becoming ever more human in appearance as the eyes move from the sides of the head to the front of the face, closed eyelids are formed, and outer ears develop further. Nail beds are beginning to form, and buds for the baby set of teeth are present. By the end of the third month, the external genitalia are clearly developed. Arms and legs grow to reach their relative length in proportion to the rest of the body, although the development of the lower limbs still lags behind that of the upper body. The brain has been growing rapidly, so that the head accounts for about one-third of the baby's sitting length, or crown-rump length. The baby's overall length is about four inches, and it weighs about 1½ ounces (40 grams). An ultrasound examination performed now may even reveal that the baby is sucking its thumb!

For a summary of your baby's growth during the embryonic period, see Table 5-2.

TABLE 5-2. SUMMARY OF GROWTH DURING THE EMBRYONIC PERIOD

Days After Conception	Length of the Embryo in Inches	Main External Characteristics
22	0.06–0.08	Embryo is still straight.
26	0.12–0.14	Embryo has become C-shaped. The arms appear as small swellings. The eyes begin to develop.
28	0.16–0.20	Hands begin to form. Legs appear as small swellings. The lenses of the eyes begin to develop.
33	0.32–0.40	Fingers are forming; the wrists and elbows become apparent. The feet begin to develop. The eyes and nostrils are clearly defined.
35	0.48–0.56	Ears begin to form; eyes become pigmented.
40	0.84–0.88	Fingers are formed and eyelids are clearly visible; toes begin to be defined.
45	1.00–1.08	The external ear becomes apparent. Toes are short and stubby; fingers become elongated.
48	1.12–1.20	The fingers and toes are clearly defined. The head, trunk, and limbs have a distinctively human appearance.

The First-Trimester Mother

"I woke up one morning and noticed that my breasts were swollen and tender. No surprise there—I was well accustomed to this particular premenstrual symptom," says Jean, a mother of three. "But then my breasts started to tingle. I said to myself in amazement, 'This isn't PMS. It feels like I'm pregnant!' I recognized that distinctive tingle from my previous pregnancy. And later that morning, a positive urine test confirmed my suspicions."

ARE YOU PREGNANT? THE EARLY SIGNS

Breast changes are indeed a common early sign of pregnancy. You may notice that your breasts become larger, firmer, and more tender, and may tingle or throb occasionally, particularly as you move into the second month. The nipples and pigmented area may darken, too.

Other early signs include fatigue, food cravings, frequent urination, and mood swings. Also, at times your heart may beat more rapidly than usual. By the end of the tenth week, your pulse increases by about fifteen beats per minute compared to your pre-pregnancy heart rate. This is because your blood volume increases by 30 to 40 percent to provide for the needs of the growing baby and placenta, as well as the increased size of your uterus and breasts. Most of this additional blood is concentrated in the pelvic area, so you may experience periods of light-headedness or may even faint if you stand up too suddenly. Nosebleeds and nasal congestion are likely to occur more frequently, too.

And of course, you may also experience that classic sign of pregnancy, morning sickness. Unfortunately, the nausea and vomiting may not be confined to the early part of the day. "It's unfair to call it morning sickness when I felt nauseated morning, noon, and night," says Jean. "And it was upsetting when people dismissed my discomfort as 'just part of being pregnant.' I was trying to eat right for my baby's sake, but how could I nourish him properly when I couldn't keep anything down? I was really worried."

NAUSEA AND VOMITING:
A SERIOUS PROBLEM

Nausea during pregnancy is believed to stem from high levels of hormones, so in this regard, it's a positive sign: It indicates that the placenta is growing and producing sufficient hormones for the pregnancy to continue. A recent study even suggested that nausea and vomiting in early pregnancy might help to ensure better growth of the placenta[1].

And morning sickness is certainly common, with an estimated 50 to 80 percent of expectant mothers experiencing symptoms not just in the morning but throughout the day, particularly in the late afternoon. Fortunately, for most expectant mothers, nausea and vomiting subside by the end of the first trimester. For about one in twenty women, though, symptoms persist in some form throughout pregnancy.

Morning sickness can be a serious problem, however—more serious than most people realize, more serious than even many doctors may realize. Extreme nausea may prevent you from eating enough to allow your baby to thrive, or even to survive. Frequent vomiting can cause you to lose the nutrients your unborn baby needs before your body has a chance to absorb them. You may also become severely dehydrated, which can increase your risk of uterine contractions and place the pregnancy at risk. Although some scientific studies have revealed little or no effect of morning sickness on rates of pregnancy complications, many other studies document an increased incidence of low birthweight and birth defects[2,3,4,5].

You can see why it's vital to your baby's positive programming that you do whatever you can to prevent such problems. The most important steps are to stay hydrated, eat foods that are easily digestible, and keep up your electrolytes by getting enough sodium and potassium. Also, look for ways to ease your nausea and vomiting. Below are some new strategies as well as time-honored techniques for overcoming morning sickness. Try some and find the ones that are most effective for you.

Take the "salty and sweet" approach. This is the newest thinking in the treatment of nausea. Foods such as potato chips, which have very little aroma but are high in salt, have been remarkably successful, particularly in combination with a sweet beverage. So try some pretzels and lemonade, or some chips and cola. Although these foods don't usually play a positive role in a healthful diet, they do have some attributes (potassium, folic acid, sodium, and of course calories). And right now, the most important thing is to eat whatever stays down. Says Jean, "I was surprised to find how well the combination of chips and cola settled my stomach in the morning. Once I was feeling better, I could go on to eat healthier foods the rest of the day."

Eat often—at least every two hours. Going too long without eating or drinking causes your blood sugar to drop, which in turn can trigger nausea, so don't let more than two hours pass without a snack or meal. Carry portable snacks such as peanut-butter crackers and a juice box in your purse or briefcase. Rebecca, a mother of two, found this strategy quite effective. "For several weeks, I vomited almost constantly. Sometimes I even had to sleep in the bathroom on a fuzzy mat all night. Then I realized that, when I got hungry, the nausea was much worse. When I ate little portions of food all day long, I felt much better."

Have a midnight or middle-of-the-night snack. If mornings are your worst time, it may help to have a slow-to-digest snack such as a grilled cheese sandwich, cereal and milk, cream-based soup, yogurt, or ice cream just before bedtime. Or set your alarm for two A.M., get up, and have a bowl of cereal with milk, then go back to bed. When you wake up in the morning, your blood sugar won't be as low as it otherwise would have been, so you shouldn't feel as nauseated.

Eat crackers in bed. If you can't bear to wake up in the wee hours, keep a box of saltines or graham crackers on your nightstand. Munch some as soon as you wake up in the morning, even before climbing out from under the covers. Or ask your partner to bring you breakfast in bed. Victoria, a mother of twins, reports, "I'd rather put up with crumbs in my sheets than have to rush to the toilet first thing in the morning. Crackers quelled that early-morning urge to throw up."

Consume protein along with carbohydrates. It is a myth that eating only fruit will ease morning sickness. Though fruit triggers a rapid rise in blood sugar that makes you feel better momentarily, soon your blood sugar falls again, leaving you even more nauseated than before. To keep blood sugar on a more even keel, be sure to eat some protein along with a carbohydrate snack.

Go for ginger. Ginger has long been used to settle the stomach. Try this recipe for ginger tea: Peel and finely dice a knuckle-sized piece of fresh ginger. Place in a mug and fill with boiling water; steep for 5 to 8 minutes. Add brown sugar to taste. Other options include ginger ale and gingersnap cookies. Abigail, a mother of two, recalls, "I drank a glass of ginger ale before getting out of bed in the morning. I also added ginger to my oatmeal at breakfast, and ate gingersnaps whenever I felt nauseous during the day. This really worked for me."

Say yes to dairy foods. Some women find that dairy products are least likely to trigger vomiting. When nausea strikes, reach for yogurt, cottage cheese, ice cream, or a milkshake.

Find beverages that ease your nausea. You and your unborn baby need at least ten cups of fluids daily, but some expectant moms find the best beverages—water and milk—are hardest to keep down. In that case, consider lemonade, ginger ale, iced tea, and cola drinks. Also experiment with temperature. Certain women think that ice-cold drinks are easiest to handle because they have less aroma. For others, beverages served warm or at room temperature work best.

"Eat" your fluids. Increase your intake of fluids with foods high in water content, such as watermelon, grapes, and apples. Suck on frozen fruit bars and Popsicles.

Take children's chewable vitamins. Prenatal vitamins often make nausea even worse. Instead, try a children's brand that contains extra folic acid, and take it at bedtime. Also try taking 75 mg of vitamin B_6 (pyridoxine) daily, which some women find relieves morning sickness.

Keep a "queasiness diary." For a few days, write down the foods you eat and try to find a pattern to your nausea. You may notice, for example, that eating fried foods sends you running for the bathroom. If so, skip the French fries in favor of a baked potato.

Avoid smells that upset your stomach. Many expectant women develop a heightened sense of smell, probably due to the higher levels of hormones such as estrogen. Aromas most likely to trigger nausea include fish, cat food, garlic, onions, coffee, perfume, and cigarette smoke. If you feel nauseated while preparing meals, order takeout or have your partner handle the cooking.

Dress comfortably. Tight clothing around the waist or neck can activate the gag reflex. Avoid turtleneck shirts and skirts or slacks with a waistband. Skip the belts. Switch from briefs to bikini underpants.

Take advantage of acupressure. Look in pharmacies or health food stores for a pair of antinausea wristbands called Sea-Bands (typically advertised as a remedy for motion sickness). Each elasticized band has a plastic button that presses on a specific spot in the wrist that is purported to ease queasiness.

None of these strategies is working for you? Don't cajole yourself into "bearing with it." Instead, call your doctor right away if:

- You haven't been able to keep any food or water down for twenty-four hours or more
- Your mouth, eyes, and skin feel dry
- You are becoming increasingly weak and fatigued
- Your ability to think clearly and to concentrate is decreasing

These are signs of serious dehydration. You may need to be admitted to the hospital to receive fluids, nutrients, and medications intravenously[6]. In fact, about 42,000 pregnant women per year in the United States are hospitalized for severe nausea and vomiting, also called hyperemesis gravidarum. The treatment you receive in the hospital should help you feel better fast—and that's exactly what your unborn baby needs most.

LOOKING AHEAD

As the first trimester comes to a close, the majority of expectant mothers find themselves feeling better every day. The fatigue and nausea that are common during the first few months of pregnancy are easing now, and you're likely to feel renewed energy. Enjoy the excitement as you switch from your regular wardrobe to maternity clothes, and share your good news with all those around you.

Food for Thought: Your Health Now and Later

The vitamin-rich diet you are eating during your pregnancy is a habit well worth keeping even after your baby is born, because it will protect your health for many years to come. For instance:

- Adequate intake of beta-carotene, a vitamin A precursor, may help prevent macular degeneration, a leading cause of blindness in adults age 50 and older. Vitamin A also may boost the immune system. Foods such as cantaloupe, peaches, carrots, spinach, fish, and dairy foods can get you to your goal of 4,000 IU per day.
- Vitamin B_6 has been shown to relieve the symptoms of carpal tunnel syndrome. To get 2 mg per day, eat bananas, brown rice, oats, whole wheat, nuts, beef, fish, chicken, and eggs.
- Adequate levels of vitamins B_{12}, B_6, and folic acid may help to improve memory and mental function later in life. Aim for

6 mcg of B_{12}, from seafood, beef liver, pork, milk, and yogurt. To get 400 mcg of folic acid, remember to eat enriched cereals, beans, asparagus, broccoli, spinach, and oranges.

Menu Ideas for These Months

The key to eating right during your first trimester of pregnancy is to choose simple foods that are easily digested. There is no magic list of foods guaranteed not to trigger nausea and vomiting, but with some experimentation, you'll find the foods that work best for you. Table 5-3 lists recommendations for foods to include and to exclude during this queasiness-prone time.

TABLE 5-3. BEST/WORST FOODS FOR THE FIRST TRIMESTER

Best Choices	Worst Choices
Bland cheese (such as mozzarella)	Broccoli
	Bell peppers
100% whole-wheat bread or toast	Brussels sprouts
	Chocolate
Cold cereal	Coffee
Cottage cheese	Mushrooms
Crackers	Onions
Fish (well-cooked)	Seasonings (including garlic, mint)
Fruit	
Juice	
Lemonade	
Lean meat (well-cooked)	
Milk	
Pasta	

Adapted from *Parenting Guide to Pregnancy and Childbirth*, by Paula Spencer, with the editors of *Parenting* magazine. New York: Ballantine Books, 1998, p. 55. Used with permission.

If you're lucky enough to sail through your first trimester with a settled stomach and an intact appetite, do remember that it's unwise to regard pregnancy as a license to eat whatever you please. Your nutrient needs increase only slightly during the first trimester, unless you were underweight before becoming pregnant. As discussed in Chapter 2, the additional 200 calories per day you need now are easily obtained through one extra daily serving each of dairy, fruits, and vegetables. The menus that follow will help you plan for the best possible first-trimester diet.

Menus for the First Trimester

FOCUS ON FOLIC ACID

Folate continues to be very important during the first trimester, as many of your baby's organs are forming and this nutrient is vital for their proper growth. Fruits and vegetables are the richest sources of this important nutrient. As outlined in Chapter 2, you should be eating at least four servings of fruit and at least four servings of vegetables each day.

An asterisk after a menu item indicates a recipe that can be found at the end of this book.

BREAKFAST IDEAS

- Date-Nut Bread* with peanut butter
- Vanilla yogurt with cherries and pecans
- Cottage cheese with raisins and granola
- Spinach and Cheese Bake*
- Fruit Crisp Delight*
- Scottish Oat Scones* with cheddar cheese slices
- Very Berry Breakfast Cake* with hard-boiled eggs
- Cheese omelet with milk

LUNCH OR DINNER IDEAS
- Old-Time Beef Stew*
- Beef and Vegetable Lo Mein*
- Hearty Bean Soup* with cheese toast
- Chicken and Dumplings*
- Orange Pork Chops* with wild rice
- Baked Ziti with Meat Sauce*
- Baked Eggplant Moussaka*
- Extra-cheese pizza with a side salad

SNACK IDEAS
- Chewy Oatmeal Cookies* with vanilla yogurt
- Whitefish spread on toasted English muffins
- Oatmeal Carrot-Cake Bread* with peanut butter
- Grilled cheese sandwich with tomato

6 ✍ THE SECOND TRIMESTER

Your goal in learning about metabolic programming is to help your baby achieve and maintain an optimal course of growth throughout gestation and into childhood. This growth is reflected not only in your baby's weight, but also head circumference, abdominal circumference, and length. The better your baby's growth is before birth, the better the chances of having a healthy childhood and adulthood.

The second trimester, defined as the fourth, fifth, and sixth months of pregnancy, presents a prime opportunity to program your child for lifelong well-being. At the end of your first trimester, your baby "graduated" from embryo to fetus status. The main difference between the embryonic and fetal periods is that now, in the fetal period, no new structures are being formed. The baby's growth is mainly in size. Yet proper nutrition—supplied through your diet, of course—is still a powerfully positive force in your baby's development.

The Second-Trimester Baby

During this trimester, prenatal testing may reveal the sex of your child—exciting information indeed, should you choose to receive it now. As a general rule, boys have a faster growth rate than girls do. Because of this difference, boys are more vulnerable to environmental factors[1,2,3].

MONTH-BY-MONTH
GROWTH AND DEVELOPMENT

No matter what your baby's sex, it's a thrill to know what's happening inside your womb at this time. If you could take a peek, here's what you would see.

The Fourth Month

Your unborn baby is about 4 inches long and weighs about 5 ounces. Lower-body development begins to accelerate.

The Fifth Month

By week twenty, your unborn baby weighs about 10 ounces and measures about 9 inches long. Lower-body development is starting to catch up to the upper body; by now your baby's head is only about one-third of his or her crown-rump length. Hair and eyebrows are visible. A soft downy growth of hair called lanugo covers the body, and a slippery white substance called vernix protects the baby's skin. Most exciting, your baby's kicks are now strong enough for you to feel!

The Sixth Month

Your baby's weight gain during this month is substantial, doubling to about 20 ounces. The baby is longer, too, achieving a length of about 12½ inches. By the end of this month the muscles have become well developed, and the baby is quite active. The respiratory and nervous systems also are developing quickly, yet are still too immature to function adequately outside the womb. The baby's skin is somewhat red and wrinkly because of the absence of fat beneath the skin. As the second trimester comes to a close, your baby's distinctive footprints and fingerprints have formed.

METABOLIC PROGRAMMING DURING THESE MONTHS

A healthy placenta is key to having a healthy baby. Yet a number of factors can interfere with proper placental growth:

- low-calorie diet
- low-protein diet
- physical stress or overactivity
- emotional stress
- smoking

These factors may cause the placenta to grow too slowly, so that it ends up small and underdeveloped. Or, strangely enough, these same factors may result in an overdeveloped placenta—one that increases its area of attachment to the uterus in an attempt to compensate for the lack of nutrients and oxygen. Poor placental development during these months can result in your child having health problems as an adult. For instance, studies have shown that a poorly developed placenta is associated with an increased risk for high blood pressure, cardiovascular disease, blood clotting problems, and diabetes later in life.

The baby's own rate of growth now is also a key factor in his or her future health. When growth slows down during the second trimester, after having been normal in the first trimester, the baby adapts by developing insulin resistance. The result is a thin baby—one whose birthweight is reduced, although body length and head circumference are normal. This child is more likely to be born early, with all the risks that entails. In adulthood, he or she will be at increased risk for non-insulin-dependent diabetes, high blood pressure, and cardiovascular disease.

Poor nutrition before birth can also adversely affect your unborn baby's future fertility. Boys who are born at a low birthweight may have a lower number of sperm-producing cells and decreased sperm output in adult life[4]. For girls, reduced growth before birth can alter hormonal patterns, causing a spectrum of reproductive and endocrine disorders after puberty. These include polycystic ovaries, infertility, acne, and other hormonal imbalances, as well as a three- to fourfold increase in her risk of developing gestational diabetes when she herself becomes pregnant[5].

An association between intelligence and birthweight has been shown in various studies. For instance:

- One Israeli study evaluated academic performance at age 17, comparing individuals who had been born small for gestational age, or SGA, to those born appropriate for gestational age, or AGA[6]. It found that SGA boys were more than twice as likely as AGA boys to have low educational attainment. SGA girls also had lower IQs than AGA girls, though the difference among girls was less pronounced.
- A study from Denmark evaluated individuals with birthweights of 4 pounds, 3 ounces (1,900 grams) to 9 pounds, 4 ounces (4,200 grams). In general, as birthweights rose, so did scores on intelligence tests[7].
- A study from the United Kingdom asked teachers to rate sixteen-year-old students. Compared to children who had been born AGA, those born SGA were less likely to be ranked in the top fifteenth percentile, and more likely to be ranked in the bottom fifteenth percentile[8].

And finally, although some children born with a low birthweight do catch up to their peers, others remain small in comparison. Studies show that adolescents and adults who were SGA at birth are significantly more likely to be shorter in height, by an average of two inches, compared to individuals who were AGA at birth[9].

NUTRITION YOU—AND YOUR BABY—NEED NOW

I tell you all this not to alarm you, but to motivate you to do everything in your power to use the effects of metabolic programming to your baby's best advantage. What you eat and drink in these months will determine, to a significant extent, the size and health of your baby at birth and beyond. Consider this:

• Babies who are well nourished in utero have significantly higher birthweights and are healthier at birth than the average baby born at the same gestational age.
• Good intrauterine growth may reduce the likelihood of premature birth. Evidence suggests that some survival mechanism, upon detecting that a baby is not growing well in the womb, may trigger labor.
• Even if born prematurely, a baby who has been well nourished in the womb has fewer illnesses and recovers from them more quickly than does an infant whose mother had an inadequate diet.

If you began taking a daily multivitamin before you got pregnant or in your first trimester, don't stop now! If you haven't been in this habit, please do start immediately. Research shows that women who take multivitamin supplements throughout their pregnancies cut the risk of early preterm delivery (delivery before thirty-three weeks' gestation) by three-fourths when they begin taking the multivitamins from the first trimester, and by half when they begin taking multivitamins during the second trimester[10]. Choose a multivitamin supplement that contains only vitamins (not minerals), and at levels equal to (not above) the RDAs for pregnancy, such as One-A-Day Essentials. Do not double up on your supplements even if you experienced severe morning sickness during your first trimester; just make sure to get the proper daily dosage now.

A second important consideration for the middle trimester is iron. As shown in Table 6-1, by this stage of pregnancy your blood volume has increased substantially over your prepregnancy levels. Red blood cells, which carry oxygen throughout the body, have increased by about 25 to 30 percent.

TABLE 6-1. THE COMPONENTS OF PREGNANCY WEIGHT GAIN

	WEEKS' GESTATION				TOTAL (LB. AND OZ.)
	10	20	30	40	
Fetus (grams)	5	300	1,500	3,400	7 lb. 8 oz.
Placenta (grams)	20	170	430	650	1 lb. 7 oz.
Amniotic Fluid (grams)	30	350	750	800	1 lb. 12 oz.
Uterus (grams)	150	350	650	1,050	2 lb. 5 oz.
Breasts (grams)	50	200	400	450	1 lb.
Blood (grams)	100	600	1,300	1,250	2 lb. 12 oz.
Extra Fluids (grams)	0	500	1,525	4,900	10 lb. 13 oz.
Muscle (Protein) (grams)	36	165	498	925	2 lb.
Body Fat (grams)	328	2,065	3,595	3,825	8 lb. 7 oz.
Total (grams)	719	4,700	7,968	17,250	
Total (lb. and oz.)	1 lb. 9 oz.	10 lb. 6 oz.	17 lb. 9 oz.	38 lb.	

Iron-deficiency anemia is a condition characterized by low levels of iron in the red blood cells. Symptoms include fatigue, lightheadedness, pallor, and shortness of breath. If untreated, anemia can adversely affect the baby's growth, and increase your own risk for complications both during and after the birth. Your doctor or midwife routinely tests your hemoglobin and hematocrit (the iron-carrying components of your blood) several times during pregnancy—typically when you begin your prenatal care, again at about twenty-six weeks, and yet again just before you deliver.

However, I do not routinely recommend iron supplements during pregnancy to treat anemia. Many women find that iron pills exacerbate nausea and vomiting. They can also lead to constipation. Furthermore, it takes more than iron to build your blood; it also takes protein, vitamin B_{12}, and other nutrients. That's why I encourage you to rely on foods rich in heme iron—lean red meats, pork, fish, poultry, and eggs—with additional iron coming from enriched or fortified grains and breads. These foods provide not only iron, but also the other blood-building nutrients that you need.

During the second trimester (and the third), be sure to include at least six servings a day of heme iron–rich foods, plus eight servings a day of enriched and fortified grains and breads. For example, you can meet those goals by including an egg and a 1½-cup serving of oatmeal with your breakfast, 2 ounces of ham on slices of whole-wheat bread at lunch, and a 3-ounce steak plus a large baked potato with dinner. (Remember to check serving sizes by referring to Table 2-2 in Chapter 2. For instance, a 3-ounce steak equals three servings of meat, while 1½ cups of oatmeal equals two servings of grains.)

Helena, a mother of two, says, "I was not used to eating much red meat. One good strategy for upping my intake was to grill steak for dinner, making enough extra to eat for lunch the next day in a cold sandwich."

DRINK WATER, WATER EVERYWHERE
Water does more than quench your thirst. It's an essential part of your daily diet. Here's why:

- Water helps dissipate the heat generated by your developing baby.
- Water lowers your risk of urinary tract infections, thereby reducing your chances of experiencing preterm labor.

- Adequate fluids help to prevent the premature uterine contractions that can trigger preterm labor.
- Mental alertness, memory, and energy levels all get a boost when you're properly hydrated.

How much water do you need? Aim for eight 16-ounce glasses of water a day. Increase that amount by an extra glass or two if:

- you are exercising regularly
- the temperature rises or the humidity falls
- you live at an altitude over 5,000 feet
- you have a history of kidney stones or urinary tract infections
- you drink more than one cup of caffeinated coffee, tea, or cola per day

Admittedly, it can be a challenge to drink this much water day in and day out. To achieve your goal, try keeping a bottle or pitcher of water with you at all times. Take a tip from Helena, who says, "Every time I thought I wanted a cup of coffee, I went and got a glass of water instead." Or try Janna's strategy: "When I get involved in my work, six hours might pass before I realize it. So I set a timer, telling myself that I had to finish eight ounces of water each hour. Having a specific plan helped me reach my quota."

The Second-Trimester Mother

Most pregnant women feel wonderful during the second trimester. The fatigue and nausea of early pregnancy have passed, and the cumbersome body of late pregnancy has not yet developed. Channel your energy in constructive ways: Take a walk each morning and evening to enhance circulation and promote relaxation. Spend more time in the kitchen preparing healthful meals and snacks. Prepare for the future by shopping for baby supplies and negotiating maternity benefits with your employer.

By the twentieth week—halfway through your pregnancy—the top of your uterus reaches to the level of your navel or just slightly below. Lying on your back while you exercise, rest, or sleep decreases blood flow to your baby as the weight of the uterus presses on the blood vessels. To enhance circulation, it's best to lie on your side.

Skin changes are common during the second trimester. A darkened line called the linea nigra may appear on your belly at this time, extending from the navel to the pubis. You also may develop a brownish discoloration on your face, called chloasma or the mask of pregnancy. Don't worry. Both are normal and will disappear after delivery. Also common are stretch marks, called striae, which appear on your abdomen due to the baby's rapid growth during these months. The streaks, which are typically pinkish or reddish, will fade to a silvery color after delivery.

If the skin on your face, hands, or body feels dry or itchy, it's a sign that you need to drink more water. It also may help to use moisturizer to relieve the dryness. If you plan to breastfeed, it's not too soon to start preparing the skin on your nipples by exposing them to the air (and sunlight, if possible), and rubbing them with a terrycloth towel after bathing.

You may find yourself sporting more varicose veins now than you did before you got pregnant. To minimize their appearance and discomfort, wear supportive stockings and elevate your feet whenever possible.

If you develop hemorrhoids, get relief by boosting your intake of fluids, fruits, and fiber. Do not use laxatives; these can cause you to lose important nutrients that you and your baby need.

Most second-trimester women generally feel warmer than before they became pregnant because of an increase in their metabolic rate, blood volume, and sweat gland activity. This last adaptation aids in the elimination of additional waste materials produced by the baby. Wear breathable fabrics like cotton, and dress in layers so you can remove extra clothing when you feel too warm. And if you and your partner are battling over the bedroom thermostat, try an electric blanket with dual controls.

WEIGHT GAIN: POUNDS AND PATTERNS

The amount of weight you gain during your pregnancy, and the pattern in which you gain it, are two very important factors influencing the growth of your baby before birth and his or her ultimate birthweight. The optimal amount of weight to gain depends on how much you weighed before you became pregnant: the lower your weight was, the more you need to gain, and the higher your weight was, the less you need to gain.

Keep this in mind: Mother Nature always invests in the best risk. If you are underweight, the initial weight you gain goes first toward correcting your own weight deficit, and only thereafter to the growth of your unborn baby. In this regard, women who begin pregnancy at a normal weight or even a little overweight have a clear advantage: The weight they gain during pregnancy goes more directly to their unborn babies. So if you were underweight before you conceived, or if morning sickness interfered with your weight gain during the first trimester, you need to work extra hard now to gain weight as quickly as possible.

Likewise, if you conceived through infertility treatments, you need to pay particular attention to your weight gain progress. If you are taking progesterone or other medications to help sustain the pregnancy, the morning sickness that other expectant mothers have already left behind may continue to affect you into your second trimester. You must replace the calories and nutrients you lose through vomiting in order to gain the weight your baby needs you to gain.

Research has shown that the pattern of weight gain may be as important as the total amount of weight gained. Try to put on the pounds as steadily as possible. The weight gained during the middle weeks of your pregnancy—from about the twentieth week to the twenty-eighth week—has the greatest effect on your baby's growth and birthweight. It's during this time that you will find that you're hungriest, and because the baby is still relatively small, you still have room for larger portions of food.

Many women have told me that they're surprised when, an hour or two after a big meal, they are ravenously hungry again. Don't feel guilty about going back to the kitchen for more! Mother Nature knows best. The biological trigger for hunger is a drop in blood sugar. What you as a second-trimester mother are experiencing is the effect of your growing baby drawing nutrients from your bloodstream, which in turn causes you to get hungry more often.

Let's look ahead to the third trimester for a moment, too. After weeks twenty-eight to thirty-two, you may find it more difficult to eat an entire meal at one time, simply because you will feel full faster. At this point, although you will still gain weight, your baby will actually be drawing upon your nutrient stores, particularly your body fat. This means that a significant portion of the weight you gain in the first and second trimesters will be converted to energy and building blocks for your baby's rapid growth during the third trimester. So don't skimp now. This is the best time to put on the pounds you need in order for your baby to thrive.

YOUR WEIGHT GAIN TARGET

Your weight gain goal is based on your prepregnancy body mass index, or BMI. As discussed in Chapter 2, BMI is a measure of your weight-for-height, with values less than 20 indicating underweight, 20 to 25 being normal weight, and over 25 being overweight or obese. Here are the optimal weight gain goals:

- If you are underweight, aim to gain five pounds or more during the first trimester, and maintain a steady rate of gain of at least one pound a week thereafter, for a total of twenty-eight to forty pounds by thirty-eight to forty weeks. This represents the pounds needed to bring you within the normal weight range for your height, plus the twenty-five to thirty-five pounds needed to allow your baby to thrive. Try to gain as quickly as possible during the first half of pregnancy, to make up for your initial weight deficit.

- If you were of normal weight before becoming pregnant, your weight gain should be about three and a half pounds during the first trimester, and about one pound a week until thirty-eight to forty weeks, for a total weight gain of twenty-five to thirty-five pounds.
- If you began this pregnancy already overweight, your weight gain should be about two pounds during the first trimester, then about two pounds a month until thirty-eight to forty weeks, for a total of fifteen to twenty-five pounds. Caution: Please do not try to maintain your current weight throughout your pregnancy, in the hopes of ending up with a slimmer figure after you deliver. This could be detrimental for your baby. Even if you were quite overweight before you conceived, you still need to gain an adequate amount of weight during pregnancy, by eating the right foods, in order to program your baby for good health.

Your prepregnancy weight doesn't tell the whole story, however. Certain women need to gain an additional three to five pounds in the first half of pregnancy in order to maximize their baby's chances for optimal growth.

- Is this your first pregnancy? The uterus of a woman who has not given birth before will not yet have been stretched. In this case, higher weight gain helps ensure better fetal growth.
- Was your pregnancy the result of infertility treatments? Though the exact reason is unclear, evidence suggests that gaining an additional three to five pounds can reduce the risk of miscarriage in pregnancies resulting from assisted reproductive technologies.

- Are you a smoker, or did you recently quit smoking? Smokers tend to have lower tissue and blood levels of many essential nutrients, and to be thinner in general. If you're still smoking, stop now. If you quit recently, good for you—but remember that your body needs time to replenish those nutrients depleted by cigarettes. Be particularly careful to eat a balanced diet, and gain an extra three to five pounds as quickly as you can.

At this point you might be wondering where all this added weight is going. If the average baby is only about 7½ pounds at birth, why do you need to gain so much above that? The answer is that many factors beyond the baby's own weight contribute to pregnancy weight gain (as shown in Table 6-1). There is your increased blood volume, additional body fluids, increased breast size, and added muscle and fat. It takes all of these ingredients for the growth of your baby to be optimal.

A word of advice: Don't weigh yourself every day; once a week is enough. Do weigh yourself at the same time of day and under similar conditions, such as first thing in the morning before you get dressed. Remember, too, that different scales report different weights, even on the same day. So don't panic if the weight you got at home is five pounds lighter than the weight at your doctor's office at your afternoon appointment. The actual number is less important than the pattern of gain over a period of weeks.

If you find yourself gaining too fast, take a hard look at your daily diet. Are you splurging on high-calorie, high-fat foods? (Anything ending in -*tos* falls into this category—Fritos, Doritos and Cheetos!) Has chocolate become one of your favorite food groups? If so, it's time to revamp your snacking habits to include more lowfat and nutritious alternatives like fresh fruits and vegetables, lowfat yogurt or cheese, and whole-grain crackers.

If you aren't gaining enough, eat more often—three meals and three substantial snacks a day. Choose foods that are nutrient rich and calorie dense, such as milkshakes, ice cream, puddings, and custards. (See the recipe section for suggestions.) If you're not able to handle larger portions, increase your fat content with foods rich in unsaturated fats, such as salad dressings, wheat germ, seeds, nuts, peanut butter, and avocados. Switch from skim to whole milk, and from lowfat to premium (16 percent fat) ice cream.

For a concise summary of weight gain guidelines during pregnancy, refer to Table 6-2.

TABLE 6-2. WEIGHT GAIN GUIDELINES
BY MOTHER'S PREPREGNANCY BMI

		First Trimester	Second and Third Trimesters	Total Gain
Underweight	BMI <20	5 pounds	more than 1 pound per week	28–40 pounds
Normal weight	BMI 20–25	3½ pounds	1 pound per week	25–35 pounds
Overweight	BMI 26–29	2 pounds	3 pounds per month	15–25 pounds
Obese	BMI >29	2 pounds	3 pounds per month	15–25 pounds

PLOTTING YOUR PROGRESS:
BETTER TOOLS THAN THE BATHROOM SCALE

Traditionally, pregnant women are weighed during each prenatal visit and that weight is recorded in the medical record. Years ago, when your own mother was pregnant with you, many doctors felt that weight gain should be limited during pregnancy. The origin of this belief arose hundreds of years earlier, when vaginal birth was difficult or impossible for any woman whose pelvis was distorted by childhood rickets. Back then, weight gain was restricted to reduce the size of the baby at birth, and improve the chances of a vaginal birth.

Today we know that weight gain is a positive, healthy sign

in pregnancy, linked to the growth of your baby before birth and his or her ultimate birthweight. But the number on the scale is not the best indicator of your nutritional status. In addition to overall weight gain, healthcare professionals often use anthropometric measures to evaluate health and nutritional status. You can take these simple, low-tech measurements at home using a tape measure.

Usually the hormonal changes of pregnancy cause you to gain weight long before your baby does. Mother Nature increases your body stores of muscle and fat to create a caloric and nutritional reserve for the second half of pregnancy, when your diet alone often can't meet your baby's metabolic demands for growth. This increase in your own body fat is a positive, healthy sign that the placenta is producing adequate amounts of hormones.

Healthcare professionals measure body fat at three sites: the upper arm, midback (at the base of the shoulder blades), and midthigh. A simple way for you to monitor changes in these areas is to measure your upper arm circumference, midway between your elbow and shoulder. Use a nonstretch tape measure, and measure consistently at the same point once a week.

An additional measurement done at each prenatal visit is an assessment of your fundal height, or the size of your uterus. While you lie on your back, the doctor or nurse measures the distance between the top of your uterus to your pubic bone; this is an indirect measure of your baby's growth. This figure, in centimeters, is roughly the same as the number of weeks of your pregnancy.

Monitoring your weight gain, charting your fundal heights, taking anthropometric measures, and estimating fetal weights from the ultrasound measurements can all help you understand your weight changes and how your baby is growing. Use Table 6-3 to keep track of your data.

As you gain weight, you'll see increases in the amount of body fat in each of the three sites discussed above. Generally, body fat increases during the first half of pregnancy, and is then mobilized during the second half. Most women find this very interesting to watch, because weight gain (as measured by the bathroom scale) and intrauterine growth (as measured by ultrasound) rapidly increase after about twenty to twenty-four weeks, while body fat (as measured by the circumference at the upper arm and midthigh) decreases after about thirty-two to thirty-four weeks. It is very satisfying to see how your body is nourishing your child even before he or she is born.

Physical Activity: What's Safe Now

Like your diet, your level of physical activity can also have a powerful effect on your baby's metabolic programming. And this, too, is a factor over which you have a lot of control—perhaps even more than you realize.

All pregnant women must be cautious when it comes to physical activity—the day-to-day kind like climbing stairs and carrying groceries, as well as the recreational choices like running or bicycling. That's because physical exertion, especially that which involves the large muscles of the back or legs, shunts blood away from your uterus, which in turn can stimulate uterine contractions. And those contractions put you at risk for preterm labor.

Stress can also have a negative effect on your unborn baby. Chronic stress increases levels of hormones called catecholamines. These hormones reduce blood flow to the uterus, interfering with placental development and fetal growth. Catecholamines can also trigger premature uterine contractions. Whether the stress is physical or mental, the effect is the same: an increased risk of having your pregnancy cut short by days, weeks, or even months. So to protect your unborn baby, follow these guidelines.

Take two naps a day. Studies show a strong connection between fatigue and preterm labor, so these naps are important. Even if

TABLE 6-3. YOUR PRENATAL RECORD

Prenatal Visit Dates													
Weeks	12	14	16	18	20	21	22	23	24	25	26	27	28
Fundal Height													
Weight Net Gain													
Weight Gain Goals													
Hemoglobin (g/dL) Hematocrit (%)													
Urine Tests Ketones Leukocytes Glucose													
Ultrasound Dates Weeks	12	14	16	18	20	21	22	23	24	25	26	27	28
Head Circumference	13 mm per week					13 mm per week				13 mm per week			
50th %ile (mm)	79	108	128	154	182	192	202	217	228	235	251	263	275
Abdominal Circumference	12 mm per week					12 mm per week				13 mm per week			
50th %ile (mm)	64	88	115	133	159	167	176	190	201	206	223	233	246
Femur Length	3 mm per week					3 mm per week				2.5 mm per week			
50th %ile (mm)	9.5	15	22	28	34	36	38	42	45	46	49	51	53
Estimated Weight	34 grams per week					90 grams per week				142 grams per week			
50th %ile (grams)	58	93	146	223	331	399	478	568	670	785	913	1055	1210

29	30	31	32	33	34	35	36	37	38	39	40
29	30	31	32	33	34	35	36	37	38	39	40
8 mm per week				7 mm per week				6 mm per week			
285	288	301	308	313	317	326	332	337	341	346	354
11 mm per week				11 mm per week				11 mm per week			
252	256	278	283	299	302	315	322	331	336	350	366
2.5 mm per week				2 mm per week				1.5 mm per week			
54.5	56	59	62	63	64	67.5	69	70.5	72	73.5	75
192 grams per week				217 grams per week				197 grams per week			
1379	1559	1751	1953	2162	2377	2595	2813	3028	3236	3435	3619

you don't sleep, the rest is beneficial. Lying down reduces cate-cholamines and also improves circulation to the kidneys and the uterus.

Lie down at the first sign of dizziness. A woozy feeling is a signal that your brain is not getting enough oxygen—which means your baby is not getting enough oxygen either. To improve circulation, get horizontal.

Lie on your side, not your back. By midpregnancy, lying on your back can decrease blood flow to the uterus and cause your baby's heart rate to drop dangerously low. It's easy for me to convince my patients of this. During a prenatal exam, we listen to the baby's heartbeat while the mother lies on her side; then we listen again as she lies on her back. Expectant mothers are always shocked at how much a baby's heart rate slows down when she's on her back—and relieved at how quickly it recovers when she turns onto her side.

Don't stand when you can sit. Women who stand for more than six hours at a time triple their risk of preterm birth. When you stand, blood vessels in the uterus are compressed against the pelvis. In an attempt to restore circulation, the uterus contracts. To prevent this, look for ways to minimize the time you spend on your feet. For instance, place a stool by the stove and sink so you don't need to stand while you cook or wash up. Set the ironing board at its lowest position and sit while you iron. Don't be shy about asking a fellow passenger to offer you his or her seat on a crowded bus. Other women in particular are usually sympathetic about the need to sit during pregnancy.

Limit stair-climbing, stooping, and bending. These activities in-volve the large lower-body muscles, and so are most likely to trig-ger contractions. To prevent this, organize household tasks to minimize trips up the stairs. On errands, take the elevator. Instead of stooping, sit on the floor to pick up clutter. Have someone else vacuum, mop, and scrub.

Avoid lifting and carrying. Weight-bearing activities cause abdominal muscles to tighten, increasing pressure on the uterus and possibly setting off contractions. Don't lift anything heavy. Instead, use a rolling basket to transport clothes to the laundry room. Find a grocery store that delivers. Put your toddler in a stroller, not a backpack.

EXERCISE DOS AND DON'TS

If you exercised on a regular basis before becoming pregnant, you know the wonderful feelings a workout brings: the sense of accomplishment in doing something good for your body, the "runner's high" triggered by the release of hormones called endorphins, and the tranquil feeling that follows.

When you're pregnant, however, your body is changing every day. While exercise offers many benefits, *you must take some special precautions now.* Anything that reduces blood flow to the placenta has the potential to adversely affect placental and fetal development—and that includes strenuous physical activity.

Lily, a mother of one, recalls, "My doctor never told me to cut back on exercise, so I continued my normal routine of an hour of aerobics four times a week. I was shocked when, at the end of my second trimester, I started having premature contractions in the middle of a workout. I was rushed straight from the health club to the hospital."

When exercising during pregnancy, moderation is the key. Even if you're in top physical condition, it's wise to cut down on the intensity and duration of your workouts. It may even be necessary to switch to a different type of workout. Here are points to keep in mind:

- Get your doctor's go-ahead before doing any exercise program.
- Switch to a less intense type of workout—walking rather than running, swimming instead of cycling, yoga in place of aerobics.
- Do not overexert yourself. Watch for the warning signs: perspiring heavily, rapid heartbeat, breathlessness, fatigue.

- Avoid activities that challenge your balance. Your center of gravity changes during pregnancy, so you're more prone to losing your balance. Also, rising levels of hormones cause your joints and ligaments to soften in preparation for childbirth. These two factors in combination leave you less surefooted than you were before pregnancy. Avoid any exercise that requires quick movements or lots of agility, or that poses a risk of falling—for instance, tennis, racquetball, volleyball, skating, skiing, aerobics, and running.
- Guard against dehydration by drinking plenty of water before, during, and after your workout.
- Do not lie on your back. After the fourth month of pregnancy, the combined weight of the uterus and the baby can block blood flow to your uterus. This in turn can lead to premature contractions and even preterm delivery.
- Maintain good posture and proper body alignment to help prevent injury.
- Moderation is especially important if you have high blood pressure, anemia, thyroid disease, or diabetes, or if your unborn baby appears to have intrauterine growth retardation.

For certain women, even moderate workouts must be avoided. The American College of Obstetricians and Gynecologists advises against exercising at all during pregnancy if you have any of the following conditions:

- an incompetent cervix
- a history of three or more miscarriages
- a history of vaginal bleeding during pregnancy
- a history of preterm labor
- a twin or supertwin pregnancy
- ruptured membranes
- cardiac disease

Working Midpregnancy

During the past forty years the number of employed women in the United States has nearly tripled, increasing from 23.2 million in 1960 to 62 million in 1996. This figure is projected to reach 70.3 million by 2005. And pregnant women make up a significant portion of this female workforce.

Not only are more expectant mothers working, they are also working longer into their pregnancies. According to a study by the U.S. Department of Census, between 1961 and 1985 the proportion of women working during the last trimester of pregnancy increased by 50 percent (from 52 percent to 78 percent), while the proportion working within one month of delivery more than doubled (from 23 percent to 47 percent)[11]. Today those figures are undoubtedly even higher.

Yet working during pregnancy, particularly during the second half of pregnancy, has been linked to several problems, including poor fetal growth, prematurity, and pregnancy-induced hypertension. Studies that examined these associations have concluded that it isn't work itself that causes problems but specific aspects of work. Top culprits include physically demanding work, prolonged standing, shift and night work, long work hours, and fatigue[12,13,14].

Women whose jobs involve a high level of physical stress run the risk of less-than-optimal placental development, which can slow down fetal growth. This is primarily due to the decreased blood flow to the uterus, and to nutrients going first to physical activity instead of to the pregnancy. Work-related mental stress, too, can increase levels of catecholamine hormones, interfering with the baby's growth and also increasing the risk of premature labor.

If you're working during your pregnancy, it's important to assess your work situation. Talk to your supervisor and ask for his or her cooperation in reducing the physical and emotional demands of your job.

- Ease the hassles associated with commuting. If your commute involves high-stress highway traffic jams, join a carpool. If your regular bus or train is always overcrowded, try traveling earlier or later so you can get a seat.
- If you work irregular hours or at night, see if you can switch to regular daytime hours.
- If your work involves standing, lifting, or carrying, ask to modify your workload or temporarily change to another position within the company.
- When work time exceeds eight hours per day or forty hours per week, risks of pregnancy complications increase. Cut back on your hours, particularly if you often feel fatigued during or after work.
- Use the phone or e-mail to communicate with coworkers, rather than walking down the hall to talk with them.
- Put a box under your desk so you can elevate your legs as much as possible.
- Build a rest period into your workday. Janna, a mother of four, says, "The smartest thing I did was to make arrangements to go home and rest for ninety minutes at midday, since I live close to the office." If going home is not an option, ask permission to lie down in the employees' lounge or rest room for thirty to sixty minutes at lunchtime each day. Then take another rest as soon as you get home in the evening.

The second trimester is a good time to plan your maternity leave. Find out what you're entitled to under the law and company policy. Generally, it's wise to take leave from work at least a few weeks before your due date, so factor that into your negotiations. Remember, if you have a difficult commute, inflexible or stressful work conditions, or pregnancy complications, you should plan to take your leave even earlier. Enlist your obstetrician's help in this. Few employers would argue with a doctor's directive stating that a leave of absence is medically necessary.

When you do go on leave, don't spend your days painting the nursery. Your unborn baby needs you to rest as much as possible, so he or she can continue to grow at an optimal rate. Once your delivery date arrives, you'll be glad to feel well-rested rather than exhausted as labor begins.

THE EXPECTANT TRAVELER

Chances are you will take at least one trip during your pregnancy, whether for work or for pleasure. The second trimester is the best time to travel, since the risk of miscarriage is over, the rate of complications is lowest now, and your energy levels are high. Check with your doctor before planning a trip, but rest assured you'll probably get the go-ahead unless you have a high-risk pregnancy or a chronic or pregnancy-induced illness. And do take the following precautions:

Identify a hospital in the area where you will be staying. If you're planning a long trip, locate several hospitals along your route. In case you do get sick during the trip, you save time and trouble by having established the location of nearby medical facilities. Carry a copy of your medical records, just in case, including laboratory tests, ultrasound reports, and prenatal records.

Buckle up. Whether traveling by car or plane, position the lap belt low on your hips, beneath rather than across your belly. In a car, the shoulder harness should go across your chest; don't tuck it behind your back.

Bring food with you. Even for short trips, it's always a good idea to have some snacks handy in case you get stuck in traffic, or your commute or errands take longer than anticipated. Stock your glove compartment or a small cooler with juice boxes, nuts, raisins, peanut butter crackers, or single-serving packs of dry cereal. Abigail, a mother of three recalls, "I always kept crackers in my purse. My husband called them 'cranky-crackers' because I'd get cranky and irritable if I hadn't eaten in a while. Those crackers

TABLE 6-4. COMPARISON OF MENU GUIDELINES FOR MOTHERS OF MULTIPLES, PRECONCEPTION, PREGNANT, AND NURSING

	PRE-CONCEPTION	SINGLETON		TWINS		TRIPLETS		QUADRUPLETS	
		Pregnant	Nursing	Pregnant	Nursing	Pregnant	Nursing	Pregnant	Nursing
Calories	2,200	2,500	2,700	3,500	3,200	4,000	3,700	4,500	4,200
Protein (grams)	110	126	135	176	160	200	185	225	210
Carbohydrate (grams)	220	248	270	350	320	400	370	450	420
Fat (grams)	98	112	120	155	142	178	164	200	187

Serving Sizes	Servings Per Day								
Dairy	4	6	8	8	10	10	12	12	14

1 cup milk
1 cup cottage cheese
1 cup ice cream
1 ounce hard cheese

Meat, fish, poultry 1 ounce	6	6	6	10	6	10	7	12	9
Eggs 1 fresh	—	1	1	2	2	2	2	2	3
Vegetables ½ cup cooked or 1 cup fresh	4	4	4	4	4	5	5	6	6
Fruits ½ cup or 1 fresh	4	4	4	7	5	8	5	8	5
Breads, grains 1 ounce, ¾ cup cooked, or 1 slice	8	8	8	10	10	12	12	12	12
Fats, oils, nuts 1 tablespoon oil, 1 pat butter, or 1 ounce of nuts	4	5	5	6	5	7	5	8	6

From *When You're Expecting Twins, Triplets, or Quads*, by Barbara Luke and Tamara Eberlein. New York: HarperCollins, 1999, p. 218.

were lifesavers when I got caught in a traffic jam or had to wait for a doctor's appointment."

Take frequent breaks. Stop the car or get up from your airplane seat at least every two hours so that you can walk around and stretch. This improves circulation and prevents leg cramps.

Hydrate before, during, and after airplane travel. Pressurized cabin air is very dry, so you are more likely to get dehydrated. Drink extra water before you board, and carry a beverage with you. You never know how long you might have to wait for the flight attendants to serve beverages.

When You're Expecting Twins (or more!)

The second trimester is when many expectant mothers get the exciting news that more than one baby is on the way. And this is happening ever more frequently, with a record-setting 118,000-plus multiples born in the United States in 1998. There are two main reasons for this surge in multiple births. First is the long-term trend for American women to postpone childbearing—and older women are naturally more likely to have multiples. The second reason is the widespread use of fertility-enhancing therapies, which greatly increase the odds of conceiving multiples.

Your nutritional requirements vary depending on the number of babies you are expecting, but in all cases your dietary needs are greater than if you were pregnant with just one baby (called a singleton). The goal when pregnant with multiples is to keep your babies growing as well as if they were singletons, even though you may deliver weeks or even months earlier. To accomplish this, you need to eat more, rest more, and gain more weight. For menu guidelines, see Table 6-4. I also recommend that you read one of our other books, *When You're Expecting Twins, Triplets, or Quads*[15].

The amount of weight you need to gain to program all your babies for optimal health depends on how many babies you're expecting, and on how much you weighed before you became pregnant. With twins, follow these guidelines:

	BY 20 WEEKS	BY 28 WEEKS	BY 36 TO 38 WEEKS
Underweight	25–35	37–49	50–62
Normal weight	20–30	30–44	40–54
Overweight	20–25	28–37	38–47
Obese	15–20	21–30	29–38

If you're expecting triplets, aim to gain at least 36 pounds by twenty-four weeks' gestation, regardless of your prepregnancy weight. With quadruplets, be sure to gain at least 50 pounds by twenty-four weeks, even if you were overweight before this pregnancy began.

KEY POINTS FOR WOMEN PREGNANT WITH MULTIPLES
- Seek out specialized prenatal care as soon as you know you're having more than one baby. Your best bet is a maternal-fetal specialist, an obstetrician with extensive training in managing the unique aspects of a multiple gestation.
- Expect to see your obstetrician more frequently than if you were carrying just one baby.
- Reduce your physical activity. If you are working, rest during your lunch hour and immediately when you get home. After twenty-four weeks, I strongly urge you to take work leave, and include two-hour naps in the morning and afternoon.
- Be aware of the warning signs of preterm labor and other potential complications. Know how to contact your doctor and hospital if you think you are experiencing problems.

- Drink at least eight 16-ounce glasses of water per day. Dehydration can trigger uterine contractions, which can lead to premature birth. Water also helps reduce the risk of urinary tract infections, another factor that increases the risk of premature birth.
- Join a mothers-of-multiples support group in your community. They provide a wealth of information as well as emotional support during this exciting but challenging time.
- Don't be bothered by thoughtless comments about your weight and size. Just tell people that your doctor says you and your babies are doing just fine!

Food for Thought: Your Health Now and Later

You're aware by now that water is vital to your unborn baby's well-being. But did you know how important water is to your own long-term health? A recent study at the Harvard School of Public Health found that people who drink 40 ounces or more of water a day cut their risk for bladder cancer in half, as compared to individuals who drink less than 16 ounces of water a day. So keep that water bottle handy, throughout your pregnancy and afterward as well.

Menu Ideas for These Months

During the second trimester, your caloric requirements increase by about 500 calories per day over your usual prepregnancy level. Those calories should come from one additional serving of dairy; two additional servings of meat, fish, or poultry; two additional servings of bread, cereal, rice, or potatoes; and one additional serving of fats, oils, or nuts. Does this sound like a huge amount of food? Remember, for instance, that a serving of meat equals one ounce—not a 16-ounce porterhouse steak. As a reminder, check back to Table 2-6.

Though the fatigue of early pregnancy has probably passed, there may be times when you need a quick pick-me-up. If you find yourself dragging with hours to go before lunch or dinner, select a snack in the 250-calorie range that provides an immediate energy boost to sustain you until your next big meal. Here are suggestions that fit the bill:

- Spread a small banana with 2 tablespoons of peanut butter
- Blend a smoothie with ½ cup nonfat vanilla yogurt, ½ cup skim milk, and ½ cup fresh fruit
- Top 8 ounces of nonfat yogurt with ¼ cup crunchy granola
- Make a trail mix with ¼ cup of nuts, ¼ cup of raisins, and ¼ cup of dried cherries
- Combine ½ cup lowfat cottage cheese with a dozen grapes and six high-fiber crackers
- Grill 2 ounces lowfat cheese on top of fresh apple or pear slices

In general, though, you can expect to feel fairly energized during your second trimester. With morning sickness behind you, you may be happy to return to your kitchen. For that reason, many of the suggested recipes for the second trimester take more time to prepare—but the delicious and nutritious results make the effort well worthwhile.

Menus for the Second Trimester

FOCUS ON IRON AND FIBER

The biggest drain on your iron stores occurs during the last trimester, so you need to stock up now. Also, as your gastrointestinal system slows down to absorb more nutrients from the foods you eat, many women get constipated. Adding foods rich in fiber to your diet, along with plenty of water, will help. Foods rich in iron include beef, poultry, pork, eggs, enriched breads and grains, nuts, beans and lentils, spinach, and wheat germ. Foods rich in fiber include fruits such as oranges, apples, raisins, and pears, and vegetables such as beans, broccoli, tomatoes, and potatoes.

An asterisk after a menu item indicates a recipe that can be found at the end of this book.

BREAKFAST IDEAS
- French toast with applesauce
- Oatmeal and scrambled eggs
- Fruitful Morning Muesli*
- Bread pudding with raisins
- Grilled cheese sandwich with Canadian bacon
- Healthy Noodle Kugel*
- Seafood Bake*
- Corn muffins with milk

LUNCH OR DINNER IDEAS
- Chicken, Lentil, and Barley Soup* with whole-wheat crackers
- Shepherd's Pie*
- Hearty Cassoulet*
- Vegetarian Chili Lasagna*

- Chicken Cordon Bleu*
- Linguine with marinara sauce
- Spinach-Stuffed Turkey Meat Loaf*
- Baked Macaroni with Peas and Ham*

SNACK IDEAS
- Baked apples with walnuts
- Quaker's Best Oatmeal Cookies* with yogurt
- Lemon Blueberry Muffins* with Muenster cheese
- My Favorite Tuna Salad* with crackers

7 ⚬ THE THIRD TRIMESTER

Nutrition is as critical for your unborn baby's development during the third trimester (the seventh, eighth, and ninth months of pregnancy) as it was in the first trimester, although for different reasons. By now all of your baby's organs are fully developed. Yet the kidneys, liver, and lungs are undergoing their periods of greatest growth, so any factors that interfere with their development now could lead, in the years to come, to chronic health problems such as asthma or hypertension.

The Third-Trimester Baby

During the final three months of pregnancy, the unborn baby is gaining weight quickly, at a rate of nearly half a pound per week. From the moment of conception to the moment of birth, he or she will have increased in size 200 billion times, to become a complex and unique individual: your baby.

MONTH-BY-MONTH GROWTH AND DEVELOPMENT

Although certain internal organs are growing most rapidly now, the nervous system and brain also continue to show significant growth during these final three months.

The Seventh Month

The baby's skin becomes less red as more fat is produced under the skin. Fingernails and toenails are fully formed, eyelids are open, eyelashes are present, and even the baby's scalp hair is well developed. The baby's bones are fully formed, but they remain soft and flexible, since the storage of both calcium and iron occurs during the last eight weeks before birth. At the end of this month, your unborn baby weighs about 3 pounds and is about 14 inches long.

The Eighth Month

By the time this month is half over, your baby has gained an additional pound of weight and has grown about 2 inches in length. At month's close, he or she weighs about 5 to 5¼ pounds and measures about 18 inches in length. The baby's skin has become smooth and pink, even in babies of dark-skinned races, since the color changes develop only after exposure of the skin to sunlight. The fine, downy growth of hair on the body has all but disappeared, and the baby has a more plump, rounded appearance.

The Ninth Month

Your unborn baby may be less active this month—it's getting crowded inside the womb! His or her skin is smooth, pale pink, and covered in waxy vernix. For babies of all races, the eyes are slate-blue now, though their true color will emerge within a few months after birth. Fingernails are firm and may extend beyond the fingertips. The breasts (in both girls and boys) may be slightly enlarged due to maternal hormones; this will gradually subside after delivery. By the time your due date arrives, your baby probably weighs 6½ to 8½ pounds and measures about 20 to 22 inches in length.

METABOLIC PROGRAMMING
DURING THESE MONTHS

In the third trimester, the growing baby normally gains weight twelve times faster than during early pregnancy. But this rate of growth can suffer a slowdown in the cases where the mother's weight gain is inadequate, her diet is low in protein or calories, she develops iron-deficiency anemia, or her physical activity and fatigue are excessive.

When this happens, the baby may adapt by sustaining brain growth at the expense of the rest of the body. This kind of disproportionate growth means the baby will probably be born at a normal birthweight, but shorter than average in length. His or her growth may continue to be poor throughout the first year of life.

If the baby is born small for gestational age, or SGA (below the tenth percentile), he or she will generally remain smaller through age four. Yet, strangely enough, this child may be predisposed to developing obesity, both in childhood and adulthood. Studies show that the percentage of body fat to muscle is higher for children who were SGA at birth[1]. These children also tend to store excess calories as fat, while protein reserves in the form of muscle remain low[2].

Before birth, SGA babies often have fetal hypoglycemia (low blood sugar). The purpose of this adaptation is to maintain the maternal-fetal glucose concentration and facilitate the transfer of nutrients across the placenta to the fetus[3]. Fetal hypoglycemia limits insulin secretion, initially increasing fetal glucose production. But this in turn causes protein to break down, limiting the unborn baby's muscle growth. After birth, this reduced muscularity in an SGA child may lead to delays in motor development. In other words, it may take longer for this baby to learn to turn over, push up, stand, walk, and explore his or her surroundings[4].

The long-term effects of the reduced muscularity and the higher percentage of body fat associated with SGA include not only a tendency toward obesity, but also an increased risk for diabetes. In studies of preadolescent children with heights below the fifth percentile, those who had been SGA at birth were significantly more likely to have abnormal insulin sensitivity[5]. During adulthood, they are also at increased risk for cardiovascular disease and hypertension.

A third-trimester slowdown in growth can also lead to organ damage. The unborn baby's liver and kidneys may fail to reach their proper size, and the blood vessels and hormonal systems that control blood pressure may be compromised. These factors lead to an increased risk for high blood pressure, high cholesterol, heart disease, and stroke later in life.

For female babies, there is an additional risk associated with slowed growth in the last trimester. Here's why: The number of immature eggs in the ovaries of an unborn baby girl reaches a peak at about the seventh month of pregnancy, and declines thereafter. These are all the eggs she will have during her entire lifespan, and each month beginning at puberty, her ovaries will release one of these eggs in preparation for a possible pregnancy. Later in adulthood, when the number of eggs remaining in the ovaries falls below a critical level, menopause will occur. Yet when an unborn baby girl's growth is impaired early in the third trimester, she is born with fewer eggs than normal. Consequently, she will enter menopause earlier in life than she otherwise would have, a situation that places her at increased risk for both heart disease and osteoporosis (the brittle-bone disease).

Nutrition Guidelines for the Final Trimester

If the information above seems disturbing, please understand that *you can do a great deal to protect your unborn baby from future health problems.* Your goal throughout pregnancy, as well as during your child's first few years of life, is to help your child achieve and maintain an optimal course of growth. Your nutritious diet is the most important tool you have through which to promote your child's positive programming.

Don't slack off on your portions even though it may be harder to eat an entire meal at one time. Your baby is taking up more room now, which means you feel full more quickly than before. You're still gaining weight, but your baby is now drawing on your nutrient stores and body fat, as well as your daily diet, for his or her own nourishment. A significant portion of the weight you gained early in your pregnancy is now being converted to energy for your baby's rapid third-trimester growth.

CALCIUM: A MIRACLE MINERAL

During the last three months in the womb, your baby's bones and teeth require a steady supply of calcium. Although this mineral has been important right from the beginning of your pregnancy, it is even more critical now. If your diet does not contain adequate amounts, calcium is mobilized from your own bones in order to meet the baby's needs[6,7]. If this occurs, your ultimate risk for osteoporosis increases significantly. The older you are, the more problematic this becomes since you have fewer years to rebuild bone density before the onset of menopause weakens your bones further.

Calcium is also an important element in the prevention of preeclampsia, a condition characterized by high blood pressure in the second half of pregnancy. This condition is discussed at greater length later in this chapter.

Your requirement for calcium-rich dairy foods increases from four servings a day during the first trimester to six servings a day in the second and third trimesters. In addition, calcium supplements provide an added measure of insurance for the proper development of your baby's bones and the protection of your own[8]. Here are suggestions for meeting your calcium needs:

• Substitute evaporated milk or calcium-fortified milk for regular milk in recipes, doubling the calcium content.
• Mix plain yogurt with dry onion soup mix to create a tasty, calcium-rich dip for vegetables.
• Try fruit-flavored yogurt on top of pancakes.
• Bake quiche for breakfast or lunch.
• Have pudding or custard for a midmorning snack.
• Choose calcium-fortified orange juice rather than regular juice.
• Choose creamy, milk-based soups rather than broth-based varieties.

TRULY ESSENTIAL: OMEGA-3 FATTY ACIDS

The omega-3 fatty acids are also vital to your diet now, for several reasons. First, they are critical to your baby's proper visual and neurologic development, which are most rapid during this period. Second, through a biochemical mechanism, they block the formation of factors that can lead to premature labor. And third, they may protect your own brainpower. During pregnancy the mother's blood level of omega-3 fatty acids drops by almost two-thirds as compared to her prepregnancy level, probably as a result of the growing baby's need for this vital nutrient. Recent studies show that the expectant mother's brain shrinks by about 3 percent during the last trimester, which may explain the memory loss that has long been associated with pregnancy. These three factors provide solid evidence for the importance of adequate omega-3 fatty acids in your daily diet.

Best sources include coldwater fish and flaxseed, olive, and canola oils. Aim to get 1,000 milligrams of omega-3 fatty acids per day. Here's how:

- Have tuna salad for lunch. A 3-ounce serving of tuna provides 500 milligrams of omega-3.
- Choose a coldwater fish such as salmon or mackerel for dinner.
- Make a snack of shrimp cocktail.
- Order anchovies on your pizza.
- Add an extra dash of oil to your salad dressing.
- Use olive oil instead of margarine on your bread.
- Sauté poultry and vegetables in canola or safflower oil rather than butter.
- Look for fresh eggs marked "enriched." These come from chickens fed fish meal or algae-enriched feed, so they are higher in the omega-3 fatty acid called DHA.

The Third-Trimester Mother

As the time of delivery approaches, your body is preparing to produce your baby's first food: breast milk. If you squeeze your breasts, you may see a small discharge of watery fluid called *colostrum*, the precursor of milk. This is normal and no cause for concern.

You also may notice a vaginal discharge that is thin, white, watery, and profuse. This, too, is normal. However, should the discharge become yellowish or thick, develop an odor, or cause any itching or irritation, it may be a sign of infection. In that case, both you and your partner should be tested and treated.

Many women in the third trimester experience heartburn, gassiness, and constipation, all of which are due to the hormonal effects of the pregnancy on the gastrointestinal tract. To alleviate these symptoms, eat small but frequent meals, drink plenty of fluids, limit fatty foods, and include ample fiber in your diet.

It's not unusual to experience a brief, occasional pain in your side, like a pulling sensation, as the ligaments supporting the uterus are stretched with the advancing pregnancy. You also may get muscle cramps or spasms in your legs, calves, or feet. These can be caused by fatigue, changing calcium levels, or the pressure of the enlarging uterus on the nerves in the pelvis. Kneading the affected area may relieve the discomfort. Also be sure to elevate your feet when resting, get some moderate exercise such as walking, and increase your calcium intake.

During these last months you may feel cumbersome and off-balance. For safety's sake, take showers instead of tub baths if you find it difficult to climb in and out of the tub without slipping. To get comfortable in bed, lie on your side (preferably the left) to promote circulation. Place one pillow under your abdomen, another between your knees, and a third rolled up at the small of your back. If you have trouble sleeping, take a warm shower before bedtime or drink warm milk with honey.

Fluid may accumulate in the tissues around your ankles and feet if you stand or walk for long periods of time. This fluid buildup is exacerbated because your uterus is pressing against the blood vessels leading to your kidneys, decreasing blood flow and interfering with the kidneys' ability to rid your body of excess fluids. To improve kidney function and alleviate swelling in the lower extremities, be sure to get plenty of rest, lying on your left side whenever possible.

By the ninth month of pregnancy, the uterus reaches to the base of the breastbone and contains nearly a quart of amniotic fluid. You may feel some shortness of breath now, as well as rapid heartbeats, because the uterus is pressing up against the diaphragm and lungs. Take care not to overexert yourself; you want to be sure that plenty of oxygen is available to your unborn baby.

SIGNS OF LABOR

Although women have been giving birth since time immemorial, scientists are still not sure what triggers labor. Various physical changes occur in concert to prepare your body for childbirth, beginning several days or even weeks before you actually deliver. When you notice the following four developments, you'll know that labor is not far off.

Lightening

About two weeks before delivery, if the baby is positioned head down, his or her head enters the pelvis, a change known as lightening. You may experience a decrease in abdominal pressure as the uterus moves away from your lungs, allowing you to breathe more deeply now. At the same time, you may feel increased pressure on your bladder and therefore may need to urinate more frequently.

Bloody Show

Very soon you may notice a gelatinous vaginal discharge (with or without streaks of blood). Called the bloody show, this is a mucus plug that has been sealing the opening to the uterus throughout your pregnancy. Its appearance indicates that the cervix, or mouth of the uterus, is beginning to thin out (efface) and open (dilate).

Rupture of Membranes

Your baby has been growing inside a membranous sac or "bag of waters." If this sac ruptures, you may feel fluid coming from your vagina, in anything from a slow trickle to a sudden gush. Often labor progresses more quickly once this occurs. This will not necessarily be your experience, however, as some women do deliver their babies with the membranes intact. For others, the membranes may rupture weeks before delivery, which increases the risk of infection. This is a very serious condition called premature rupture of membranes, or PROM. It's vital that you call your doctor immediately if you even suspect that your membranes have ruptured.

Uterine Contractions

You've probably been feeling some contractions throughout your pregnancy. Called Braxton-Hicks contractions, these are normal. Yet they differ from true labor contractions in that they are irregularly spaced (as timed from the beginning of one contraction to the beginning of the next); they are brought on by fatigue, dehydration, or physical activity; and they disappear with rest and hydration.

True labor contractions are different. When your body goes into normal full-term labor, the initial contractions may be mild, short, and irregular—but as labor progresses, contractions become stronger, closer together, and more regular. Typically the contractions occur at regular intervals of five minutes or less, with each contraction lasting about thirty to sixty seconds, and they continue regardless of what you do.

Be sure you understand completely what your doctor wants you to do when you suspect that labor is beginning. Have your suitcase packed ahead of time so you won't be worrying about what to take to the hospital. Line up childcare in advance for your other children, if necessary. And arrange for your partner or another driver to be ready at a moment's notice to take you to the hospital when the time comes. When these details are worked out ahead of time, your childbirth experience is much calmer and more enjoyable.

Recognizing Complications

The majority of expectant mothers sail through all three trimesters of pregnancy with no medical problems whatsoever. However, it's wise to be familiar with the warning signs of complications. The earlier a problem is detected, the more likely it can be treated before serious consequences develop.

GESTATIONAL DIABETES

You will be tested for gestational diabetes around the beginning of your third trimester using the oral glucose screening test described in Chapter 4. Your risk for developing this condition is higher if you:

- are over age 30
- are overweight
- have a family history of diabetes
- have a history of miscarriage or stillbirth
- have given birth to a baby weighing more than nine pounds
- are expecting twins, triplets, or quadruplets

The body requires insulin, a hormone produced by the pancreas, to pull carbohydrates into the cells for use as energy. By the sixth month of pregnancy, the baby is growing so fast that the mother must make extra insulin. Yet at the same time, the placenta produces hormones that interfere with the action of insulin. When the insulin supply cannot keep up with the demand, the mother's blood sugar levels rise and she becomes temporarily diabetic. This condition is called gestational diabetes.

If gestational diabetes is not controlled, the unborn baby's nervous system may be affected because it lacks sufficient glucose. One warning sign of this risk is the presence of ketones in your urine, an indication that your diet does not contain enough carbohydrates. Long-term studies have found an association between ketones in the expectant mother's urine and reduced IQ during childhood[9,10,11,12,13,14].

Gestational diabetes may also cause the unborn baby to grow too large, increasing the risk of trauma at birth and perhaps necessitating a cesarean delivery. And immediately after birth, the baby may suffer from hypoglycemia (low blood sugar) and other metabolic and respiratory problems.

To guard against gestational diabetes, remember that your need for carbohydrates is now double what it was before you got pregnant. Aim to get 250 to 312 grams of carbohydrates per day. Find out whether any members of your extended family have diabetes or developed gestational diabetes during pregnancy; if so, tell your doctor. Also be alert for these warning signs:

- excessive thirst
- increased frequency and volume of urination
- constant fatigue
- recurrent vaginal yeast infections

If you do develop gestational diabetes, your obstetrician may recommend that two new members join your healthcare team: a physician who specializes in diabetes, and a registered dietitian. You will need to follow a special diet in which your consumption of carbohydrates is evenly spaced throughout the day. In fact, the diet plan for gestational diabetes is very similar to the program outlined in this book, except that simple sugars (table sugar, jellies, jams, syrups, cookies, candies, pies, and cakes) are not allowed. In most cases, diet therapy is effective in controlling blood glucose levels, although some women may need insulin injections as well.

If you develop gestational diabetes, your dietitian may recommend a food system called Exchange Lists to be used in planning your meals. This system groups together foods that are alike. For each of your meals, you select a certain number of items (or exchanges) from each of the six food categories. This makes it easy to plan meals that offer plenty of variety, yet contain approximately the same number of calories and the correct amount of carbohydrate, protein, and fat. The Exchange Lists are shown in Table 7-1.

TABLE 7-1. EXCHANGE LISTS FOR MEAL PLANNING WITH DIABETES

Starch Exchanges

1 piece bread

1 tortilla

6 crackers

½ cup pasta, corn, potatoes, or
hot cereal

½ cup beans, peas, or lentils*

⅓ cup rice

¾ cup flaked cereal

Fat Exchanges

1 tsp. margarine, oil, mayonnaise,
or butter

1 tbsp. diet margarine or low-fat
mayonnaise

1 tbsp. salad dressing

2 tbsp. low-fat dressing

⅛ of an avocado

20 small peanuts

8 large olives

2 tbsp. sour cream

1 slice bacon

Milk Exchanges

SKIM OR VERY LOWFAT MILK EXCHANGES

1 cup skim, ½% fat, or 1%
fat milk

1 cup buttermilk

1 cup nonfat or lowfat sugar-
free yogurt

¾ cup plain nonfat yogurt

LOWFAT MILK EXCHANGES

1 cup 2% fat milk

¾ cup plain lowfat yogurt

WHOLE MILK EXCHANGES

1 cup whole milk

1 cup kefir

Meat/Meat Substitute Exchanges

VERY LEAN MEAT EXCHANGES

1 oz. fish or shellfish

1 oz. chicken or turkey breast

1 oz. fat-free cheese

1 oz. lunch meats
(with 1 gram or less of fat
per ounce)

¼ cup nonfat or lowfat cottage
cheese

½ cup cooked beans, peas, or
lentils*

LEAN MEAT EXCHANGES

1 oz. round, sirloin, or
flank steak

1 oz. pork tenderloin, ham, veal,
or leg of lamb

1 oz. dark-meat chicken, no skin

1 oz. cheese
(with 3 grams or less of fat
per ounce)

1 oz. lunch meats
(with 3 grams or less of fat
per ounce)

*Beans, peas, and lentils count as a starch and a lean meat exchange.

MEDIUM-FAT MEAT EXCHANGES

1 oz. most other beef

1 oz. mozzarella cheese

1 oz. cheese
(with 5 grams or less of fat per ounce)

1 egg

1 oz. dark-meat chicken, with skin

1 oz. salmon or tuna in oil (drained)

1 oz. ground turkey

½ cup tofu

HIGH-FAT MEAT EXCHANGES

1 oz. spareribs

1 oz. sausage

1 oz. regular cheese

1 oz. hotdog or lunch meats
(with 8 grams or less of fat per ounce)

Fruit Exchanges

1 medium fresh fruit

½ banana

12 cherries

15 grapes

½ cup canned fruit, unsweetened

Vegetable Exchanges

½ cup cooked vegetables

½ cup vegetable juice

1 cup raw vegetables

From "Exchange Lists for Meal Planning," American Diabetes Association and American Dietetic Association, 1995.

Key Points for Women with Gestational Diabetes

- Now it's more important than ever to eat three meals and three snacks a day, each with a balance of proteins, carbohydrates, and fats, particularly foods rich in omega-3 fatty acids.
- A program of regular, moderate exercise (such as walking or leisurely swimming) helps to maintain stable blood glucose levels, an important factor for the growth of your unborn baby.
- Include fiber-rich foods in your diet to further stabilize blood glucose.
- Monitor your blood glucose level on a regular basis, as directed by your diabetes healthcare team.
- After delivery, gestational diabetes disappears. Do be alert for the reappearance of warning signs, however, since women who've

had this pregnancy complication are more likely to become diabetic later in life.

PREECLAMPSIA

Preeclampsia is a serious complication affecting about 7 percent of all expectant mothers, typically in the second half of pregnancy. It is characterized by a rapid rise in blood pressure, the presence of protein in the urine, sudden and extreme weight gain, and fluid retention. The cause of preeclampsia is not known, but it's more likely to develop in women with preexisting hypertension, in women who are pregnant for the first time, and in women expecting twins, triplets, or quadruplets. After delivery, blood pressure returns to normal.

Be alert to the signs and symptoms of this dangerous complication:

- Severe or constant headache
- Sudden weight gain of more than one pound a day
- Blurred vision or dark spots in front of your eyes
- Pain in the upper-right quadrant of your abdomen
- Swelling of your face and hands

Some scientists believe that preeclampsia may be related to a deficiency of calcium during pregnancy. Research has shown that the regular intake of dairy foods throughout pregnancy can cut the risk for preeclampsia by as much as 40 percent[15]. Other studies have shown a reduction in preeclampsia with calcium supplementation, alone and in combination with linoleic acid[16,17,18]. Recent research has linked dietary deficiencies of riboflavin to preeclampsia[19]. The lesson: *Proper nutrition reduces your risks of serious pregnancy complications right up through your final trimester.*

PREMATURE LABOR

When labor starts before the end of the thirty-seventh week of pregnancy, it is considered preterm. Preterm labor can lead to premature birth, which occurs in about 10 percent of births in the United States every year. As the single most important problem in pregnancy, premature birth is one of the leading causes of disability. Half of all deaths that occur before the first birthday are due to pregnancy-related factors—and nine out of ten of these deaths are due to prematurity and its complications.

Premature babies, or preemies, are more than just small. They are developmentally unprepared for life outside the womb. If they survive, they are more likely to have problems growing and developing normally. Children who were born prematurely may have respiratory problems during childhood, as well as a higher incidence of learning disabilities and problems with speech, hearing, and vision. The more premature the infant is, the more severe the complications are likely to be.

Prematurity has long been a perplexing problem for obstetricians and pregnant women alike. There is no single cause and no single solution. Many factors contribute to a woman's risk of delivering prematurely, although the same risk factor may not have the same effect in two different women. Women at higher risk include those who:

- have a history of premature labor or premature birth
- are pregnant with multiples
- have complications of the cervix or uterus, such as incompetent (weak) cervix or uterine fibroids
- have placental complications, such as placenta previa
- develop vaginal or urinary tract infections
- have premature rupture of the membranes
- were underweight before they conceived and have not gained enough weight during pregnancy

- have chronic hypertension
- have a pregnancy complicated by birth defects

If premature labor is stopped early enough, delivery can be postponed, buying your baby valuable time to grow and mature. Even a few extra days inside the womb can make an important difference in your child's health at birth and beyond, particularly as it gives your doctors the needed time to administer steroids that will improve your baby's lung function at birth and reduce the respiratory complications of prematurity.

This is why it's so important that you be aware of any premature contractions you may experience. If this is your first pregnancy, appreciating what a uterine contraction feels like is difficult. Not all women feel contractions in the same way. Ask any two women about their labor experience and you will probably hear two completely different stories. For one woman, the contractions she felt before and during labor may have been very intense and severe. For another woman, contractions may have been moderate or even mild, no worse than monthly menstrual cramps. And even if you have given birth before, each pregnancy is different; your contractions this time may be quite different from your previous experience. So keep in mind that uterine contractions, particularly premature ones, may not be painful.

Uterine contractions are usually perceived as a heaviness in the abdomen or as pain in the mid- to lower back, accompanied by a tightening of the uterus. Some women say the tightness feels like a fist squeezing inside their belly. When you feel this heaviness or pain, you should place your hands on your abdomen, at the top of your uterus, to determine if these sensations are accompanied by a tightening or hardening of your uterus. When you squeeze your biceps to "make a muscle" in your arm, you can feel the muscle go from being loose to being hard. When your uterus contracts, you can feel the tightening the same way.

After you detect uterine contractions, you should determine what you were doing when they started. The circumstances that trigger uterine contractions can vary greatly from woman to woman. For example, for one woman it may be walking for long periods while shopping, carrying a child in her arms, or vacuuming rugs. For another woman it might be standing on the train during her commute home, carrying groceries, or hanging wallpaper. For a third, it may be an argument with a coworker or a heated discussion with her in-laws over baby names. Regardless of the circumstances, it is important for you to:

- Recognize that uterine contractions are occurring.
- Identify what activity brought on the contractions.
- Stop that activity and sit down or, preferably, lie down on your left side.
- Drink several glasses of water, since dehydration can also cause contractions.
- Time the contractions from the beginning of one to the beginning of the next.
- If the contractions do not subside, call your doctor and follow his or her advice.

Along with uterine contractions, there are several other warning signs of preterm labor. Study this list:

- rhythmic or persistent pelvic pressure
- menstrual-like cramps, with or without diarrhea
- sudden or persistent low backache
- vaginal discharge, particularly that which changes in color, consistency, or amount

Because these symptoms can be vague, they are all too easy to dismiss. "For weeks I had felt frequent yet painless contractions, which I assumed to be Braxton-Hicks. That pelvic pressure I experienced (particularly when tired), I interpreted as a normal discomfort of pregnancy. My persistent lower backache, I attributed to muscle strain," explains Jean, a mother of three. "Yet if I had recognized these symptoms for what they really were, I might have received medical attention in time to halt preterm labor. Instead, my baby was born at thirty-one weeks, weighing just three pounds, and he spent a month in the neonatal intensive care unit. He's healthy now, but it was a very rough start."

I would like to add one more point to the list above (which your obstetrician should discuss with you in detail): If you have any intuition, premonition, or "funny feeling" that something just isn't right, let your doctor know without delay. Sometimes a vague impression is the only warning you'll get. I'm reminded of the day a patient at my clinic came in for a routine checkup at thirty weeks. She said, "I've been feeling kind of down lately—achy and depressed, nothing more. I wasn't even going to bother mentioning it, but my mother insisted I tell you." We did a pelvic exam and also monitored her for contractions, and sure enough, she was experiencing preterm labor. We immediately took steps to stop the labor, and succeeded in postponing delivery for an additional seven weeks. Yet if that woman hadn't mentioned the way she'd been feeling, her preterm labor would have progressed, and she would have delivered much sooner.

Be sure to call your doctor, day or night, if you experience even a single symptom. It's far better to be told it's a false alarm than to ignore an alarm that's real.

IF YOU NEED BED REST

Many complications of pregnancy share a common treatment: bed rest. Staying horizontal for a few weeks (or even months) can do a number of positive things for your baby and for you. For instance, it can:

• conserve your energy so that more of what you eat goes directly to promoting your baby's growth

- increase circulation to the uterus, thus providing additional oxygen and nutrients to your unborn baby
- improve blood flow to your kidneys, which helps to eliminate excess fluids
- minimize blood levels of catecholamines, the stress hormones that can trigger contractions
- limit your physical activity, thereby reducing contractions
- take pressure off your cervix
- reduce the strain on your heart

The least restrictive form of bed rest is called modified bed rest. Typically, this means you stay in bed for two hours every morning and again every afternoon, as well as all evening and all night. You may be allowed brief excursions outside the house, as long as you avoid overexertion. Diane, a mother of twin girls, recalls, "I was warned not to do any lifting or vacuuming during my hours out of bed. That was hard as a woman, not to be able to take care of my house or do the cooking. Dr. Luke kept reminding me that the dust didn't matter—I could dust after the babies were born."

If your doctor puts you on strict bed rest, it means you must spend almost all your time lying down. Be sure to make arrangements for maintaining your diet. And keep your calorie count up, even if inactivity suppresses your appetite. Victoria, a mother of two, says, "My husband put a little refrigerator next to our bed and kept it stocked with nutritious foods. My mom brought me food, too. She wanted her grandchild-to-be to grow big and strong!"

Just because you are stuck in bed doesn't mean life has to stop. Plan your day and your activities, and the time will pass more quickly. If possible, I suggest setting up two beds—one in the bedroom and the other on a sofa in another part of your home. Stock each area with a phone and phone book, a good reading lamp, books, magazines, catalogs, pens, and paper. Work on embroidery or quilting. Earn some continuing education credits. Get a laptop and hone your computer skills. Organize your recipes or sewing patterns. Start your Christmas shopping or order your baby's layette from catalogs or the Internet. Once you put your mind to it, you'll be surprised to discover how many things can be done right from bed. And always remember that the most important thing you're doing as you lie there: You're helping your baby to grow.

Food for Thought: Your Health Now and Later

Those omega-3 essential fatty acids that are so important to your unborn baby's development are also a safeguard for your health as you age.

- In a twenty-year follow-up of middle-aged men from the Netherlands, Finland, and Italy, the regular consumption of fatty fish (which are rich in omega-3 fatty acids) was found to be associated with a 33 percent reduction in the risk of death from coronary heart disease[20].
- In a study of 1,569 women, the consumption of broiled or baked fish twice or more per week was associated with a 43 percent reduction in the risk for rheumatoid arthritis[21].

Menu Ideas for These Months

Most women don't feel like cooking much during these last months. Your best strategy is to conserve time and energy by using simple menus for your meals. Since calcium and the essential fatty acids are the key nutrients during the third trimester, I've included lots of delicious menus that fit the bill. As Victoria says, "Crock-Pot meals were wonderful during my third trimester. I'd prepare roast beef with carrots and potatoes and other veggies, and it was enough to make three meals out of one cooking session. My other quick and easy favorite was spaghetti with tomato sauce and meatballs."

A word to the wise: Stock up now on kitchen essentials like paper towels and dishwashing detergent. Space permitting, fill your pantry with cereals, soups, canned vegetables, dried fruits, pastas, and sauces. When you do find extra energy for culinary pursuits, consider casseroles and other dishes that can be prepared now and frozen. In the busy weeks after the baby is born, you'll be very glad to have your cupboards and freezer already stocked with heat-and-eat meals.

Menus for the Third Trimester

FOCUS ON CALCIUM AND OMEGA-3 FATTY ACIDS

This trimester your need for foods rich in calcium and the omega-3 fatty acids is greatest. Calcium is found in dairy foods as well as eggs, beans, peanuts, tofu, potatoes, spinach, and salmon (with bones). Good sources of omega-3 fatty acids include eggs, seafood and fish, and safflower, canola, flaxseed, and soybean oils.

An asterisk after a menu item indicates that a recipe can be found at the end of this book.

BREAKFAST IDEAS

- Shrimp Egg Foo Yung*
- Asparagus omelet with sliced pears and cheese
- Cottage cheese with peaches and pineapple
- Vegetable Quiche*
- Bagels with cream cheese and lox
- Spanish omelet and whole-wheat toast
- Egg salad with cinnamon raisin toast
- Blueberry muffins with milk

LUNCH OR DINNER IDEAS
- Tuna Casserole*
- Caesar Pasta Salad*
- Shrimp and Noodles with Peanut Sauce*
- Peanut Pork Chops* with green beans
- Chicken and Yam Stew* with steamed spinach
- Mushroom-Spinach Bake*
- Vegetable Tofu Stir-Fry* with steamed rice
- Sesame Tuna* with coleslaw

SNACK IDEAS
- Yogurt with graham crackers
- Fish Chowder*
- Lemon Yogurt Cookies* with milk
- Toasted English muffins with farmer cheese

8 ❧ THE "FOURTH TRIMESTER" AND YOUR BABY'S FIRST YEAR

You've met the challenges of pregnancy and childbirth, and now you hold your precious newborn in your arms. Congratulations! In the happy but hectic times to come, remember that your goal is to assure that your child's first weeks and months outside the womb continue a pattern of healthy programming. Yes, that's right—*metabolic programming does not stop at the moment of birth*. Your child's brain, respiratory system, and pancreas are all still developing, while your own body is undergoing important changes that allow it to continue nourishing your newborn—which is why the postpartum period is sometimes called the "fourth trimester." You can protect your child's future health by providing the best possible nourishment, monitoring his or her progress in growth and development, guarding against infection, and avoiding environmental toxins.

Metabolic Programming in the First Year

Was your baby born well grown and full-term (at thirty-eight weeks' gestation or later)? If so, fantastic! He or she has reaped the benefits of positive programming before birth, and is off to a great start.

Or was your baby born prematurely? Symmetrically small? Thin but with a normal birth length and head circumference? Short but with a normal birthweight and head circumference? Such situations indicate that growth was less than optimal before birth, but don't be discouraged. Your baby has the most to gain from the metabolic programming processes that occur in early childhood. The positive steps you take in the next months and years can go a long way toward safeguarding your child's health for decades to come.

YOUR BABY'S BRAIN

Your baby's brain and nervous system continue to grow and develop throughout early childhood. This means they are still vulnerable to damage—including subtle changes in structure and chemistry, as well as a resetting of hormonal controls—from poor nutrition. Depending on the timing and the specific types of cells affected, such damage can lead to lowered intelligence, cerebral palsy, vision problems, behavioral disorders, schizophrenia, or clinical depression[1,2].

Fortunately, the opposite also holds true: Optimal nutrition now is key to preventing problems and assuring proper development of the brain. Good nourishment in early childhood can even help a child overcome some of the effects of inadequate nutrition he or she received in the womb.

Positive Programming for Your Baby's Brain

What's the best way to encourage proper brain development during the first year? Undoubtedly, the answer is breastfeeding. The human brain is composed of about 60 percent fat. The omega-3 fatty acid DHA is the most abundant kind of fat present in the brain—and it is also the most abundant fat present in breast milk. Infant formula does not contain this vital nutrient. This is one reason I strongly urge you to breastfeed your newborn in order to provide the very best nourishment for your child's growing brain. (See "Why Breast Is Best" later in this chapter.)

THE RESPIRATORY SYSTEM

A baby is born with only about half the number of alveoli (the air cells of the lungs, where gases are exchanged in respiration) that he or she will eventually need, so lung development continues for the first two years after birth. If the development of alveoli is impaired—due to inadequate nutrition or respiratory infections, for instance—the lungs cannot grow to their proper size, nor can they function as well as they should. The possible result: chronic respiratory problems that persist throughout childhood and adulthood.

The risk is greatest in the following situations:

- *Among children with a low birthweight or other indication of poor prenatal growth.* When lung development has been compromised before birth and development continues at a reduced rate during infancy, there's a much higher likelihood of chronic bronchitis.
- *Among boys.* Due to differences in the pattern of early lung growth, boys generally have a larger lung volume but more narrow airways than do girls of similar age and stature. In infancy, boys suffer more severe lower respiratory tract infections than girls do. And in early life, boys are more likely to be hospitalized with bronchiolitis (inflammation of part of the airway) due to their smaller airway size[3].
- *Among children exposed to secondhand smoke.* When someone lights up, other people in the room breathe in the smoke that wafts from the burning cigarette, as well as the air that the smoker exhales after each puff. This is called "passive smoking." When a baby is a passive smoker, his or her developing lungs become damaged, thereby increasing the probability of chronic

respiratory problems throughout childhood and adulthood. And far worse, the baby's risk for sudden infant death syndrome rises significantly, particularly if he or she was born prematurely or at a low birthweight[4,5,6].

Positive Programming for Your Baby's Lungs

There are a number of simple steps you can take to program your baby for a lifetime of healthy lung function:

- Never let anyone smoke in your house. Lily, a mother of one, recalls, "My father was a chain smoker, and as a child I always seemed to have some kind of chest cold or cough. Back then, no one made the connection between passive smoking and respiratory problems. I was determined not to let the same thing happen to my son, so I was very strict about forbidding friends and family to smoke in our home."

- If you are a former smoker who quit during pregnancy, do yourself and your baby a big favor: Don't start smoking again! Even if you vow not to smoke when your baby is in the room, the contaminated air lingers long after the cigarette has gone out.

- To avoid infections, limit your baby's exposure to people who are sick. Ask friends not to visit your home if they are not feeling well. If your caregiver has a cold, use a backup baby-sitter for a few days. When a family member is ill, minimize the time that person spends with the baby. When you're feeling under the weather, be sure to wash your hands before touching the baby, and try to avoid breathing on him or her.

- Keep your home as free as possible from respiratory irritants such as dust. Change the air filters in your heating and cooling systems frequently. Do not use baby powder on or near your child.

THE PANCREAS

The pancreas, you'll recall, plays a primary part in the regulation of carbohydrate metabolism. During infancy the cells of the pancreas continue to differentiate as they take on specific functions within the organ. The hormone insulin is secreted by the part of the pancreas known as the beta cells of the islets of Langerhans.

If a baby's prenatal growth slows during the second or third trimester, the pancreas will be adversely affected. If nutrition during infancy continues to be poor, the consequences include damage to the structure and function of the beta cells of the islets of Langerhans. This changes the way the tissues of the body respond to insulin, placing the child at highest risk for developing the insulin resistance syndrome: diabetes, hypertension, and abnormal blood lipids.

Positive Programming for Your Baby's Pancreas

Because the pancreas is still growing after your baby's birth, the window of opportunity has not yet closed. Good nutrition during infancy can still protect the pancreas and help your baby to achieve his or her optimal growth. Breastfeeding, along with the careful introduction of nutritious solid foods at the appropriate times, can ensure that your baby receives the best possible nourishment.

Feeding Your Baby

Your baby should receive only breast milk, infant formula, or a combination of the two for the first six months after birth. Breast milk or formula should continue to be your baby's primary food until he or she is consistently eating table food, which usually occurs between eight and twelve months of age. Do not switch from breast milk or formula to cow's milk until your baby is one year old.

Most babies do not need any additional vitamins or minerals

beyond those supplied by breast milk or infant formula. Your pediatrician may recommend additional iron if your baby has low iron stores or anemia, while vitamin D supplementation may be necessary for infants who are not exposed to adequate sunlight.

WHY BREAST IS BEST

There's very little you need to do to prepare for nursing, since Mother Nature has done the preparation for you. What you need most is encouragement, along with this one piece of vital information: With very few exceptions, *human milk is the optimal food for all infants,* especially those who are sick or premature. I strongly recommend that you breastfeed your baby for at least a year, and that breast milk be your baby's only food for the first six months. Here's why.

Breast milk boosts your baby's brainpower. Research shows that breastfed children have higher IQs. Studies of eight-year-olds and eighteen-year-olds alike have demonstrated a substantial superiority in intelligence and academic success among those who had been breastfed[7,8]. These findings have been confirmed recently in studies of premature infants: Upon reaching school age, preemies who had received breast milk outperformed those who had received formula[9].

Asthma is less common among children who were breastfed. Asthma is the single most prevalent cause of childhood disability, and over the past twenty-five years the rates of childhood asthma have more than doubled[10]. Children at highest risk include those whose mothers smoke, those who were born prematurely, and those who weighed less than 5½ pounds at birth. Recent research shows that breastfeeding exclusively for at least the first four months after birth can significantly reduce a child's risk of asthma at age 6[11].

Nursing reduces a baby's risk of infection and allergies. Colostrum, the early milk your breasts produce in the first several days after childbirth, helps to guard against jaundice, assists in clearing meconium from your baby's system, and provides antibodies that protect against infection. Also, studies show that infants who are exclusively breastfed during the first six months of life have significantly lower risks for illnesses, including ear infections, respiratory infections, and diarrhea, as compared to babies who are bottle-fed[12, 13, 14,15].

Nursing stimulates an infant's visual development. Studies show that breastfed children generally have better visual perception than do their formula-fed nursery mates.

Breast milk is more satisfying for your baby. The unique composition of breast milk cannot be duplicated by any infant formula. Each feeding provides foremilk, a watery milk that quenches your baby's thirst, followed by the creamier hindmilk that satisfies hunger.

Nursing is also beneficial for the mother. Breastfeeding increases the mother's levels of the hormone oxytocin, which reduces postpartum bleeding. Oxytocin also helps shrink the uterus from its weight of 2¼ pounds immediately after childbirth, to only 2 ounces at six weeks postpartum. Women who breastfeed return to their prepregnancy weight sooner and also lose more body fat, particularly if they nurse for at least six months[16,17].

Despite these clear advantages, currently only about half of all infants in the United States are breastfed. Of these, only 40 percent are exclusively breastfed for four months, and only 5 percent receive breast milk through the first year[18].

Why so few? First, because many women are under the misconception that they can't make enough milk to satisfy their baby. In truth, this problem is extremely rare. Milk production is a supply-and-demand process: The more your baby suckles, the more milk you will make. To get nursing mothers off to a good start, many hospitals encourage them to give the first feeding in the recovery room, immediately after delivery. Ask a nurse, lactation consultant, or midwife about any problems or concerns you may have. Another good strategy is to feed your baby on demand—whenever he or she seems hungry, rather than according to some preset schedule. This helps both of you to establish a pattern and lays the groundwork for successful breastfeeding.

The second reason women hesitate to breastfeed, or discontinue breastfeeding after just a couple of months, is that they plan to return to work. However, many companies nowadays encourage nursing employees to make use of special private areas for pumping and storing breast milk. This is an excellent option. Your caregiver can use your expressed milk in your absence, and you can continue to enjoy nursing your infant when you're at home.

DIET TIPS FOR BREASTFEEDING MOTHERS

Your diet is the key to producing the quantity and quality of breast milk needed in order for your baby to thrive. It's simple to make the necessary adjustments in what you eat, because a nursing mother's diet is very similar to your pregnancy diet, but with more dairy foods and fewer servings of meat.

Plan to consume about 250 calories more per day than you did before you were pregnant. Even if you are overweight, you should take in at least 2,000 calories a day while nursing. Now is not the time to diet! But don't worry about getting your figure back: Breastfeeding mothers lose more body fat—particularly from the hips—than mothers who choose to bottle-feed their babies, because milk production uses up some of the calories that were stored as body fat during pregnancy.

Refer to Table 8-1 for a comparison between the nutritional requirements for breastfeeding and non-nursing mothers. This may seem like a lot of food, but remember how serving sizes were defined in Chapter 2—for instance, one serving of meat equals one ounce, not a half-pound slab of steak.

To simplify your food selection process even further, I've translated these recommendations into a day's worth of menus in

**TABLE 8-1. NUTRITIONAL REQUIREMENTS AND MENU GUIDELINES
FOR BREASTFEEDING AND BOTTLE-FEEDING MOTHERS**

Nutritional Requirements	Bottle-feeding	Breastfeeding
Calories	2,000	2,700
Protein (20–25% of calories)	100–125 g	135–169 g
Carbohydrate (40–50% of calories)	200–250 g	270–338 g
Fat (30–40% of calories)	67–89 g	90–120 g
Menu Guidelines (servings per day)		
Dairy	3	8
Meat, fish, or poultry } Cooked beans Cooked lentils	4–6	6
Eggs	0–1	1
Vegetables	3–4	4
Fruits	3–4	4
Breads, cereals } Pasta, rice, potatoes	6–8	8
Fats, oils, nuts	2–3	5

Table 8-2, again comparing the needs of nursing and non-nursing mothers. Chances are, your appetite will match your nutritional needs. "I did feel hungrier when nursing, compared to the end of pregnancy when I didn't have any room for food," says Victoria, a mother of two.

Be sure to get enough protein, iron, and calcium in your diet. I say this more as a safeguard for your own health than for your baby's. The content of protein, carbohydrate, and fat in breast milk is amazingly constant, and varies only slightly based on the

TABLE 8-2. COMPARISON OF A TYPICAL MENU FOR
BOTTLE-FEEDING VERSUS BREASTFEEDING MOTHERS

	BOTTLE-FEEDING	BREASTFEEDING
Breakfast	Scrambled egg with butter	+ 1 oz. grated
	Whole-wheat toast with	cheese
	all-fruit jam	
	Orange and grapefruit sections	
	Milk, 1% or skim	Substitute whole milk
Snack		+ Lowfat yogurt
Lunch	Tuna melt with 2 oz. tuna and	
	1 oz. cheese on rye with	
	lettuce and tomato	
	V-8 vegetable juice cocktail	substitute whole milk
Snack	Lowfat yogurt and fresh	+ Graham
	fruit shake	crackers
Dinner	Grilled salmon, 4 oz.	
	Mixed salad with olive	+ 1 oz. grated
	oil and vinegar dressing	cheese
	Steamed squash	
	Steamed asparagus	
	Baked potato	
	Iced tea	Substitute whole milk
Snack	Rice pudding with raisins	+ Oatmeal cookies

mother's diet. So while your baby is likely to do all right even if your diet isn't ideal, your own health and energy may suffer.

Breast-milk content does vary for certain nutrients, however, depending on the mother's diet. That's why your breastfeeding baby needs for you to eat plenty of the following:

- *Omega-3 fatty acids.* While the quantity of fat in your breast milk remains fairly constant no matter what you eat, the type of fat does depend on your diet. In order for your breast milk to be rich in the omega-3 fatty acids your baby needs for proper visual and neurologic development, your diet also must be rich in these fatty acids. Boost your intake by eating seafood, fish (particularly salmon and tuna), fresh eggs enriched with vitamin E and omega-3 fatty acids, and oils such as canola, safflower, walnut, and olive.
- *Zinc.* If your diet is deficient in zinc, your breast milk will be too—and this mineral is vital to your baby's neurologic development. Good sources of zinc include beans, whole grains, nuts, beef and lamb, poultry, eggs, and yogurt.
- *Iodine.* In order for your baby to get the iodine necessary for proper thyroid function, you must eat foods that contain this important mineral. Best sources include fish and seafood, bread, milk, and iodized salt.

It's not just the helpful nutrients you ingest that wind up in your breast milk. When you drink caffeine or alcohol, when you take medications, when you smoke a cigarette—the toxins in all these things find their way into your breast milk and into your baby. Just as you were careful during pregnancy about what you put into your body, so must you take care while nursing. Everything you ingest may also affect your baby, and often more adversely. Here are guidelines:

- If you drink coffee, limit yourself to no more than three cups per day, or switch to decaffeinated.
- Alcohol enters your breast milk and interferes with protein synthesis, which in turn affects your baby's growth. Ideally, you should avoid alcohol until after your baby is weaned. If you do drink, limit yourself to one drink or less per day. To reduce the amount of alcohol that enters your breast milk, be sure not to

drink on an empty stomach. Also, nurse your baby before you have that glass of wine, not afterward.

- Do not smoke.
- Before taking any prescription or over-the-counter medication, check with your doctor, and remind him or her that you are breastfeeding. (Recently, the FDA determined that nasal decongestants and appetite suppressants containing phenylpropanolamine are associated with an increased risk of stroke, particularly in young women. These medications are no longer being sold; you should discard any that you may have in your medicine cabinet.)

IF YOU CHOOSE BOTTLE-FEEDING

Have you decided to supplement your nursing with an occasional bottle, to switch from breast to bottle before your child's first birthday, or to forgo breastfeeding altogether in favor of infant formula? Then rest assured that generations of children have grown healthy and strong with this type of first food.

Most formulas are derived from cow's milk. If your baby has allergies or a sensitive stomach, however, he or she may do better on a soy-based or protein-hydrolysate formula. Be aware, too, that the infant formulas currently available in this country do not contain the critical nutrient DHA, although in Europe infant formulas have been supplemented with long-chain polyunsaturated fatty acids (including DHA) for nearly a decade. This issue is under review by the Food and Drug Administration, and new regulations for manufacturers are expected in the near future. In the meantime, ask your pediatrician about the advisability of supplementing your baby's diet with this vital nutrient.

Most infant formulas come in three types. Ready-to-pour is the most convenient but also the most expensive. Liquid formula concentrate is cheaper, yet must be mixed with sterilized water, and any unused portion has to be promptly refrigerated. Powdered formula is the least expensive option. An opened can of powder does not require refrigeration, but it too must be combined with sterilized water and mixed well to prevent lumps.

Formula should be gently warmed before being given to your baby. Never heat a bottle in the microwave oven; too many babies have had their mouths badly scalded this way. Instead, warm the bottle by placing it in a bowl of hot tap water for a few minutes. Before serving, test the temperature on the inside of your wrist to make sure it is warm but *not* hot.

One other note of caution: *Never put your baby to bed with a bottle.* If milk is allowed to pool in the baby's mouth during sleep, serious tooth decay can result. There is also the danger that the baby could choke, should he or she bite through the rubber nipple while you are not there to immediately handle the emergency.

FEED YOUR SOUL

However you choose to nourish your baby, don't forget to nourish your own body and spirit too during these exciting but exhausting weeks. Let someone else clean your house, buy the groceries, and do the laundry while you focus on enjoying and getting to know your baby. Your body needs rest in order to heal from the challenges of pregnancy and childbirth, and fatigue increases your risk of postpartum depression[19]. So instead of calling the office or writing thank-you notes while your baby sleeps, use this time to take a relaxing, warm shower or, better yet, a nap. You deserve it!

Starting Solid Foods

Starting solid foods is an exciting milestone, but please do not rush toward it. When solid foods are introduced too early, the baby is more likely to develop allergies and respiratory illnesses later in childhood. Studies also link the early introduction of solid foods to an increase in body fat and blood pressure during childhood[20]. On the other hand, when solid foods are delayed too long, there's a risk of iron-deficiency anemia and slowed growth.

For babies born at full term (after thirty-seven weeks' gestation), solid foods should be introduced at about six months of age. If your baby was premature, your pediatrician may recommend delaying solid foods until what would have been the six-month mark had the baby not been born early—in other words, six months after your due date.

STEP-BY-STEP GUIDELINES

Generally, before a baby can learn to swallow solid foods, he needs to be able to sit up with minimal support, follow the spoon with his eyes, and open his mouth when he sees food coming. Introduce only one new food at a time, to make sure your baby has no allergic reactions. Refer to Table 8-3 for the nutritional requirements for good health and growth during the first year.

TABLE 8-3. DIETARY REQUIREMENTS DURING INFANCY

	BIRTH TO 6 MONTHS	7 TO 12 MONTHS
Calories	650	850
Protein	13 g	14 g
Vitamins		
Vitamin A	375 μg RE	375 μg RE
Vitamin B_6	0.1 mg	0.3 mg
Vitamin B_{12}	0.4 μg	0.5 μg
Vitamin C	40 mg	50 mg
Vitamin D	5 μg	5 μg
Vitamin E	4 mg	6 mg
Thiamin	0.2 mg	0.3 mg

	BIRTH TO 6 MONTHS	7 TO 12 MONTHS
Riboflavin	0.3 mg	0.4 mg
Niacin	2 mg	4 mg
Folate	65 μg	80 μg
Pantothenic Acid	1.7 mg	1.8 mg
Biotin	5 μg	6 μg
Choline	125 mg	150 mg
Minerals		
Calcium	210 mg	270 mg
Fluoride	0.01 mg	0.5 mg
Iodine	40 μg	50 μg
Iron	6 mg	10 mg
Phosphorus	100 mg	275 mg
Magnesium	30 mg	75 mg
Selenium	15 μg	20 μg
Zinc	5 mg	5 mg

RDAs and DRIs from the Food and Nutrition Board of the National Academy of Sciences, 2000.

The best way to meet the requirements in Table 8-3 is by following these steps:

Step 1: Iron-fortified infant rice cereal mixed with breast milk or formula should be your baby's first solid food. Do not move on to step 2 until your baby is well established on infant cereal, taking at least a half-cup per day, divided into two or more meals. Continue giving your baby iron-fortified cereal throughout the first year, and even into the second year.

Step 2: Cooked fruits and vegetables can be pureed or fork-mashed. If you make your own, be careful to use very clean produce and cooking utensils, and do not add any salt or sugar.

Step 3: Finger foods come next, usually breads and cereals. When your baby can grasp foods and bite and chew reasonably well, it's time to offer soft and cooked foods that the baby can pick up with his or her fingers. Again, be sure that the baby's portion has no added salt or sugar.

Step 4: Meats that are ground or finely diced are generally introduced when the baby is eight to twelve months old. By this time, your baby has reduced the amount of breast milk or formula he or she is consuming, and needs an alternative protein source.

Step 5: Pasteurized whole milk can gradually be substituted for breast milk or infant formula when your baby has reached one year of age and is eating about three ounces of solid food, three times a day. At mealtimes, offer the milk in a lidded cup rather than a bottle. (It's fine, and in fact quite beneficial, to continue breastfeeding at other times of the day for as long as you and your baby are both content to do so.)

In Table 8-4, I've listed some nourishing foods appropriate for older infants, along with the daily requirement for various nutrients. But don't be too concerned if your child doesn't meet the recommended numbers every single day. A well-balanced diet is determined by what the baby eats over the course of several days or a week. And remember that serving sizes are smaller for children than for adults. For a toddler, a serving of fruits or vegetables equals one to two tablespoons. A bread or cereal portion is about one-quarter the size of an adult portion.

FOOD SAFETY FOR THE FIRST YEAR

Food safety is another issue that needs your particular attention as your baby makes the transition to table foods. Food poisoning and choking are serious dangers. To reduce the risks to your child, take the following precautions[21]:

TABLE 8-4. SUGGESTED FINGER FOODS FOR OLDER INFANTS (6–12 MONTHS)

NUTRIENT	DAILY REQUIREMENT	FOOD (AMOUNT)	NUTRIENT CONTENT
Vitamin A	375 µg	Cheerios (½ cup)	188 µg
		Winter squash (¼ cup)	120 µg
		Cooked spinach (¼ cup)	370 µg
Vitamin B$_{12}$	0.5 µg	Beef tenderloin (½ oz.)	0.35 µg
		Ground beef (½ oz.)	0.25 µg
		Yogurt (¼ cup)	0.35 µg
Vitamin C	50 mg	Orange juice (2 oz.)	25 mg
		Kiwi fruit (½ medium)	38 mg
		Pink grapefruit (¼ medium)	24 mg
		Strawberries (¼ cup)	22 mg
		Cantaloupe (½ cup)	34 mg
Vitamin E	6 mg	Sweet potatoes (½ medium)	2 mg

NUTRIENT	DAILY REQUIREMENT	FOOD (AMOUNT)	NUTRIENT CONTENT
Vitamin E (continued)		Peanut butter* (1 tablespoon)	3 mg
		Rice cereal (½ cup)	5 mg
Calcium	270 mg	Mozzarella cheese (1 oz.)	147 mg
		Yogurt (¼ cup)	104 mg
		American cheese** (1 slice)	124 mg
		Cottage cheese** (½ cup)	63 mg
		Broccoli (½ cup)	47 mg
Iron	10 mg	Rice cereal*** (1 oz.)	3.5 mg
		Ground beef (1 oz.)	0.9 mg
		Tuna, canned in water (1 oz.)	0.4 mg
		Baked potato (½ medium)	1.4 mg

*Be sure to dilute with formula or breast milk to make it easier to swallow.
**Calcium-fortified brands (like Light n' Lively) have twice the calcium content.
***Made with whole milk.

- Do not give honey or corn syrup to any child less than one year old. These foods may contain botulism spores that are harmless to older children and adults, but can cause serious illness in a baby.
- Do not offer nuts, seeds, raw carrots, raisins, popcorn, jellybeans, or any round hard candy until your child is three years old.
- Proper food preparation can reduce the risk of choking. Slice

a hot dog lengthwise into strips rather than into circles. Cut grapes into quarters. Cook carrots until soft. Remove all bones from fish.

- Mix peanut butter with milk, applesauce, or mashed banana to make it less sticky and easier to swallow. Spread a small amount on a cracker or soft bread; do not let your child eat it straight from a spoon.
- Always be present when your child is eating. Do not allow other children to supervise your baby's meals.
- Keep your child in the high chair during meals and snacks. Choking occurs more often when children eat on the run.
- Keep mealtimes calm. There's a greater risk of inhaling food when a child is laughing or shouting.

First-Year Growth and Development

A baby is born with a number of reflexes that indicate growth of the nervous system. The baby will grasp your finger strongly (the grasp reflex); he or she will turn his or her face to the side when touched (the rooting reflex); and he or she will automatically start sucking when something touches his or her lips (the sucking reflex). All of these reflexes are adaptations to life outside the womb.

A newborn baby's head may appear elongated from the molding that occurs during a vaginal birth. This is normal. The head returns to a more rounded shape within a few weeks.

Newborns can breathe only through their noses, and they can do so while eating. Any nasal congestion, therefore, causes a baby difficulty in both breathing and eating. You can help by softening mucus inside the nose with over-the-counter saline nose drops, then suctioning it out with a suction bulb.

There are several signs that indicate when a child is thriving. Here's what to watch for:

- *Wet diaper count.* During the first day or two after birth, your baby may have only one or two wet diapers. But by the fourth or fifth day, and each day thereafter, you should expect to see at least six to eight wet cloth diapers or five to six wet disposable diapers (which are more absorbent and therefore may become saturated more slowly).
- *Bowel movements.* In the first several days after birth, a newborn passes a tarry black stool called meconium. By the third day of life, your baby should be producing two to five bowel movements daily.
- *Behavior and appearance.* A baby who is thriving has good color and skin tone, is active and alert, wakes up for feedings, and is generally content after being fed.

TRACKING YOUR BABY'S GROWTH

The most important sign of a thriving baby, of course, is his or her rate of growth. The average baby born at forty weeks' gestation weighs about 7½ pounds and is about 22 inches in length, although there is wide variation that is still considered normal. Typically a baby loses about 5 to 10 percent of his or her body weight, approximately 6 to 10 ounces, in the first few days after birth. Your baby should be back at his or her birthweight within two weeks, and may experience a growth spurt—and appetite boost—around three weeks of age. From that point on, the baby should gain weight steadily at a rate of about an ounce a day, or two pounds a month, for the first six months. As a general rule, a baby doubles his or her birthweight by the age of four months, and triples it by the first birthday. Breastfed babies may weigh slightly less than their formula-fed peers from eight to eleven months of age, but there will be no significant differences at later ages.

A considerable amount of the weight your infant is gaining now is in the form of body fat, which for babies is very healthy.

The average newborn has about 11 percent body fat, whereas by one year of age, this figure has more than doubled, to about 24 percent.

In Chapter 4, I provided tables of the tenth, fiftieth, and ninetieth percentiles of growth for head circumference, abdominal circumference, femur length, and fetal weight as a means to monitor how your baby was growing before birth. Now that your baby is here, it's much easier to track his or her growth. At the end of this chapter are the newest growth charts from the National Center for Health Statistics of the Centers for Disease Control and Prevention, which were released in June 2000. These are the same national growth charts that your child's pediatrician uses. By plotting all aspects of your child's growth, you can better monitor progress over time. There are separate charts for boys and for girls, and each includes percentiles from birth to thirty-six months for the following:

- weight-for-age
- length-for-age
- weight-for-length
- head circumference-for-age

For the majority of children born light or short for gestational age, catch-up growth occurs within the first three to nine months of life[22,23]. By late adolescence, less than one out of ten of these children are shorter than their peers[24]. Symmetrically small babies (those with a slower rate of growth starting early in pregnancy) are most likely to remain shorter throughout childhood.

Children have a predetermined pattern or trajectory of growth, both before and after birth, which is defined by a combination of genetics and environment. During even a brief illness, your child's appetite is likely to drop, and this may be reflected in a leveling off or even a slight fall in weight. But with recovery, appetite increases and growth returns to normal, often making up for any losses. Do not worry about these minor setbacks. Most important is the overall pattern of growth, along with the growth attained by the first birthday. *Do keep track of your child's growth,* and discuss it with your pediatrician. Remember, your baby's growth this year is a vital component of his or her metabolic programming. The sooner any slowdown is noticed, the sooner it can be remedied.

Growth and the Loving Touch

Many studies over the years have shown that babies who are raised in a more stimulating environment have better growth and development. The difference is particularly pronounced among babies who were born prematurely or small for gestational age[25,26,27].

Many simple forms of stimulation can help your baby to grow and develop—being rocked, massaged, and held. Studies from neonatal intensive care units have revealed that development improves when babies receive "kangaroo care" by being snuggled skin-to-skin against a parent's chest. Talking, reading, and singing to your baby can also enhance development. So take every opportunity to interact with him or her. You'll be doing your child a world of good—and enjoying yourself immensely in the process.

Food for Thought: Your Health Now and Later

Breastfeeding is best not only for your baby's future health, but also for your own long-term well-being.

- Women who breastfed a baby have a reduced risk of ovarian cancer[28].
- Premenopausal breast cancer is less common in women who have breastfed. Studies show that women who breastfed for ten to fifteen months have a 43 percent lower risk of breast cancer.

Women who breastfed at least two babies reduced their risk of breast cancer by 33 percent[29,30].

- Are you concerned that breastfeeding may increase your risk of eventually developing osteoporosis? It's true that studies have documented a significant loss of bone mass during breastfeeding, particularly in the spine and hip joint, in the range of 4 to 5 percent. But after weaning, bone mass increases by more than this amount—so the bone loss is normal, temporary, and more than compensated for in the long run[31,32,33,34,35,36].

- Research has shown that the body's ability to repair itself is linked to nutritional status. Poor nutrition may adversely affect tissues that must last a lifetime, such as the lens of the eye and the collagen and elastin in muscles[37]. This in turn can cause premature aging. The lesson? Good nutrition is a veritable fountain of youth.

Menu Ideas for These Months

If you're breastfeeding, you need about 250 extra calories beyond your prepregnancy requirements. Your diet should be similar to the one you followed during pregnancy, but with more dairy foods and less meat. Listed below are menus and recipes that provide the nutrients and calories nursing moms need to produce premium milk. If you're bottle-feeding, check out the menus and recipes designed to help you achieve your prepregnancy weight, heal from pregnancy and childbirth, and maintain your energy.

Menus for the "Fourth Trimester"

FOCUS ON OMEGA-3 FATTY ACIDS, ZINC, AND IODINE
Because the type of fat in your breast milk reflects the fats in
your diet, you should include ample amounts of foods rich
in omega-3 fatty acids, such as fish and seafood, and canola,
safflower, and olive oils. The amounts of zinc and iodine in
breast milk are also influenced by the foods in your diet.
Rich sources of zinc include beans, whole grains, nuts, beef,
pork, poultry, eggs, and yogurt. Iodine is found in breads,
fish and seafood, and milk.

An asterisk after a menu item indicates a recipe that can
be found at the end of this book.

BREAKFAST IDEAS
- Salmon-Noodle Bake*
- Vanilla yogurt with walnuts and wheat germ
- Ham and cheese omelet
- Fruit Crisp Delight*
- Whitefish spread on toasted sesame bagels
- Spinach and Cheese Bake*
- Oatmeal with raisins
- Wholesome Apple-Raisin Muffins* with milk

LUNCH OR DINNER IDEAS
- Cashew Chicken*
- Creole Shrimp Bake*
- Salmon Fishcakes*
- Turkey Breast with Cherries and Pecans*
- Orange Pork Chops*
- Bowties and Chicken with Peanut Sauce*
- Sylvia's Seafood Sauté*
- Grilled salmon with potatoes au gratin

SNACK IDEAS
- Granny Smith apple slices with peanut butter
- Deviled eggs with Ry-Krisps
- Daybreak Date Bread* with farmer cheese
- Healthy Noodle Kugel*

CDC Growth Charts: United States

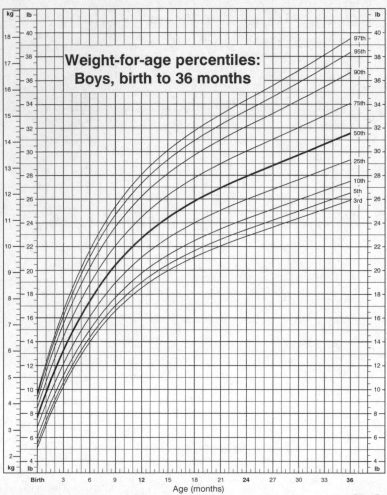

Weight-for-age percentiles:
Boys, birth to 36 months

SOURCE: Developed by the National Center for Health Statistics in collaboration with
the National Center for Chronic Disease Prevention and Health Promotion (2000).

CDC Growth Charts: United States

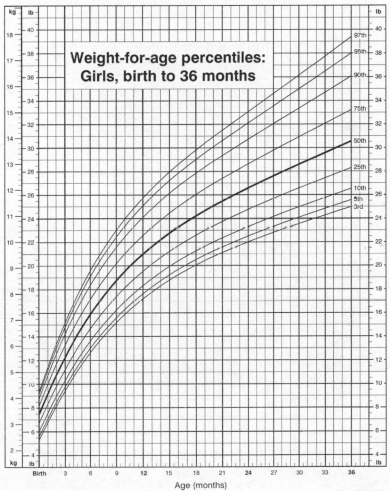

Weight-for-age percentiles:
Girls, birth to 36 months

Age (months)

SOURCE: Developed by the National Center for Health Statistics in collaboration with
the National Center for Chronic Disease Prevention and Health Promotion (2000).

CDC Growth Charts: United States

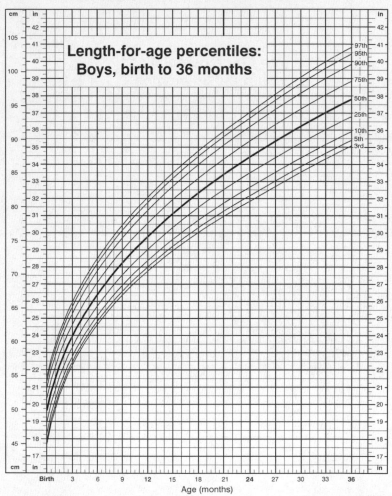

**Length-for-age percentiles:
Boys, birth to 36 months**

SOURCE: Developed by the National Center for Health Statistics in collaboration with
the National Center for Chronic Disease Prevention and Health Promotion (2000).

CDC Growth Charts: United States

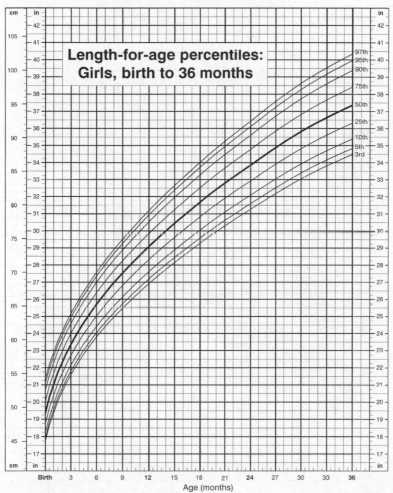

**Length-for-age percentiles:
Girls, birth to 36 months**

SOURCE: Developed by the National Center for Health Statistics in collaboration with
the National Center for Chronic Disease Prevention and Health Promotion (2000).

CDC Growth Charts: United States

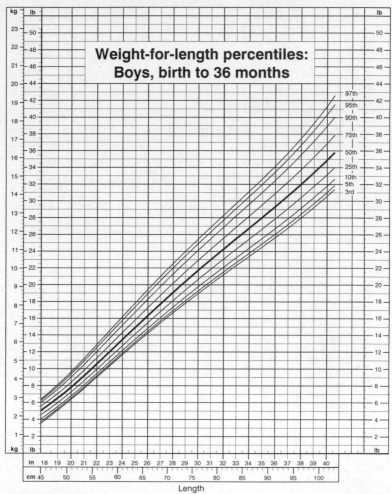

Weight-for-length percentiles: Boys, birth to 36 months

Length

Revised and corrected June 8, 2000.

SOURCE: Developed by the National Center for Health Statistics in collaboration with the National Center for Chronic Disease Prevention and Health Promotion (2000).

CDC Growth Charts: United States

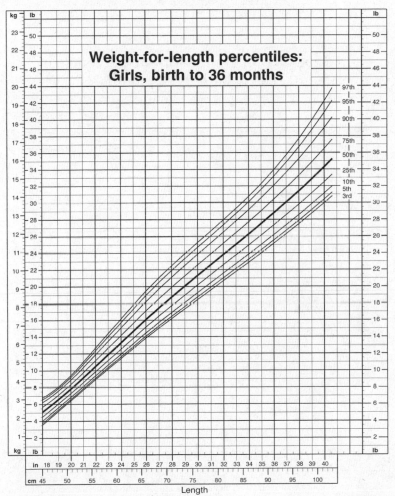

Weight-for-length percentiles: Girls, birth to 36 months

Revised and corrected June 8, 2000.
SOURCE: Developed by the National Center for Health Statistics in collaboration with
the National Center for Chronic Disease Prevention and Health Promotion (2000).

CDC Growth Charts: United States

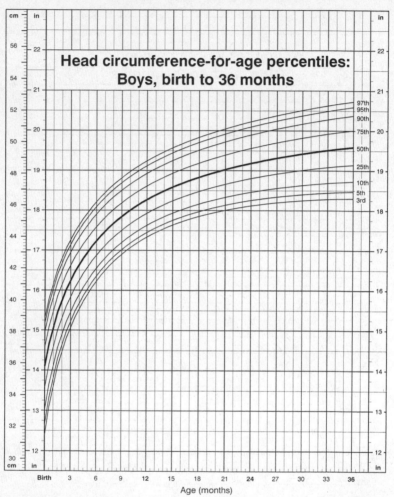

Head circumference-for-age percentiles: Boys, birth to 36 months

Age (months)

SOURCE: Developed by the National Center for Health Statistics in collaboration with
the National Center for Chronic Disease Prevention and Health Promotion (2000).

CDC Growth Charts: United States

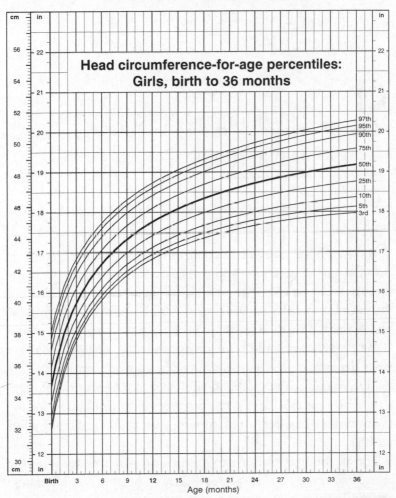

Head circumference-for-age percentiles:
Girls, birth to 36 months

SOURCE: Developed by the National Center for Health Statistics in collaboration with
the National Center for Chronic Disease Prevention and Health Promotion (2000).

9 ❧ CHILDHOOD, ADOLESCENCE, AND BEYOND

Children born today can expect to have longer, healthier lives than any generation before them. Life expectancy today is seventy-four years for men and eighty years for women. That's a full decade more than it was for children born fifty years ago, and fifteen years more than for those born sixty years ago[1].

Yet your own child's longevity and the quality of those years depend in great part on his or her growth during the formative years of childhood and adolescence. These growing years represent your final opportunity to lower your child's risk for many chronic diseases, programming your child for lifelong good health.

For all children, the keys to optimal growth and development are a healthy diet, regular physical activity, healthy lifestyle habits, and sufficient rest. Such measures help to prevent illness and obesity in childhood, and reduce the risk of cardiovascular disease, hypertension, diabetes, infertility, osteoporosis, and even cancer (see Table 9-1).

TABLE 9-1. LEADING RISK FACTORS FOR THE MAJOR ILLNESSES

	Diet	Smoking	Excessive Alcohol Use	Obesity	Central Adiposity	Physical Inactivity	Estrogen Deficiency
Cardiovascular Disease	•	•		•	•	•	•
Cancer (general)	•	•		•		•	•
Lung		•					
Breast	•		•	•	•	•	
Colorectal	•	•	•			•	
Gyn*				•			
Osteoporosis	•	•	•			•	•
Diabetes	•			•	•	•	
Infertility	•	•	•	•			•

*Cervical, endometrial, ovarian.

Childhood Growth and Development

Childhood growth typically follows predictable patterns. By around age 2, weight gain generally levels off to about five pounds per year for boys and about four pounds a year for girls; this rate of growth does not begin to climb again until adolescence. By age 4, a child's height is approximately double his or her birth length. The percent of body fat in a healthy child typically increases from 11 percent at birth to 24 percent by one year of age, then falls to 21 percent by age 2, and to about 18 percent by age 3. The majority of children who had been born small for gestational age are, by age 4, within a normal range of height and weight; only about one in ten remains small or short[2].

The newest growth charts for boys and girls ages 2 to 20, which were recently released by the National Center for Health Statistics of the Centers for Disease Control and Prevention, can be found at the end of this chapter. Similar to the charts presented earlier for children under age 3, these charts can help you track your child's growth, notice any slowdown, and seek medical advice if necessary. The charts include percentiles for the following measures:

- weight-for-age
- stature-for-age
- weight-for-stature
- body mass index-for-age

You may be surprised to learn that *children grow the most during sleep*. Adequate sleep, in fact, may even help to slow the aging process[3,4]. That's why sufficient rest is vital to your child's development. Here are the average daily requirements during early childhood, based on age[5].

- A one-year-old needs fourteen hours of sleep, including eleven and a half hours at night and two and a half hours of nap time.
- A one-and-a-half-year-old needs thirteen and a half hours of sleep, including eleven and a half hours at night and two hours of nap time.
- A two-year-old needs thirteen hours of sleep, including eleven and a half hours at night and one and a half hours of nap time.
- A three-year-old needs twelve hours of sleep, including eleven hours at night and one hour of nap time.
- A four-year-old needs eleven and a half hours of sleep at night.
- A five-year-old needs eleven hours of sleep at night.

Nutritional Requirements in Childhood

As a parent you can do a great deal to increase the odds that your child will experience optimal growth and continued positive programming. In the early years, you have near complete control over your child's diet. Later on, as your youngster becomes more independent, the good habits you instill early on will help your child make wise food choices throughout life.

The earlier you begin, the easier it is to encourage healthful eating. Abigail, a mother of three, says, "I give my toddler a fruit with breakfast, and a vegetable with lunch and dinner. I also make sure he gets enough protein. As soon as he was interested in what we were eating, we fed him from our plates so he'd get used to eating normal foods. Now he's a great eater—not at all fussy about trying new things, and perfectly content to have a banana instead of a cookie."

Remember, though, that children do have different nutritional requirements from adults: Children need more energy, carbohydrates, and fats. And because kids can't eat the large volume of food that adults can, they need foods that are higher in calories and nutrients.

TABLE 9-2. DIETARY REQUIREMENTS DURING EARLY CHILDHOOD

	1 to 3 years	4 to 8 years
Calories	1,300	1,800
Protein	16 g	24 g
Vitamins		
Vitamin A	400 µg RE	500–700 µg RE
Vitamin B_6	0.5 mg	0.6 mg
Vitamin B_{12}	0.9 µg	1.2 µg
Vitamin C	15 mg	25 mg
Vitamin D	5 µg	5 µg
Vitamin E	6 mg	7 mg
Thiamin	0.5 mg	0.6 mg
Riboflavin	0.5 mg	0.6 mg
Niacin	6 mg	8 mg
Folic acid	150 µg	200 µg
Pantothenic acid	2 mg	3 mg
Biotin	8 µg	12 µg
Choline	200 mg	250 mg
Minerals		
Calcium	500 mg	800 mg
Fluoride	0.7 mg	1 mg
Iodine	70 µg	90–120 µg
Iron	10 mg	10 mg
Phosphorus	460 mg	500 mg
Magnesium	80 mg	130 mg
Selenium	20 µg	30 µg
Zinc	10 mg	10 mg

Recommended Dietary Allowances (RDAs) and Dietary Reference Intakes (DRIs) from the Food and Nutrition Board of the National Academy of Sciences, 2000.

In early childhood, you can't just go by the USDA Food Pyramid, since it is geared toward individuals ages 7 and older. For that reason, I've given you a chart of the nutrient requirements for children ages 1 to 3, and for children ages 4 to 8, in Table 9-2.

In brief, each of your child's meals should include the following:

- protein such as fish, poultry, eggs, or beans
- bread, pasta, and/or cereal
- fruits or vegetables, or both
- milk

To help you make sure your child meets his or her nutritional requirements, I've translated the RDAs for children into servings in Table 9-3. (Keep in mind that serving sizes are typically smaller for younger children, averaging about half the portion for an older child or adult.)

TABLE 9-3. MENU GUIDELINES FOR YOUNG CHILDREN

NUMBER OF SERVINGS PER DAY BY AGE GROUP

	1 to 3 years	4 to 8 years
Milk group	2 servings	3 servings
	4 oz. milk	6–8 oz. milk
	2 oz. yogurt	6–8 oz. yogurt
	2 oz. cottage cheese	3–4 oz. cottage cheese
	1 oz. hard cheese	1½–2 oz. hard cheese
Meat group	2 servings	3 servings
	1 oz. meat, fish, or poultry	1½–2 oz. meat, fish, or poultry
	2 oz. cooked beans	3–4 oz. cooked beans

	1 to 3 years	4 to 8 years

Bread group	4 servings
	½ slice of bread
	¼–⅓ cup packaged
	   or cooked cereal
	¼ cup cooked pasta,
	   rice, or potatoes
		6 servings
		½–1 slice of bread
		¾ cup cereal
		½ cup cooked pasta,
		   rice, or potatoes

Vegetable group	3 servings ¼ cup cooked ½ cup fresh	5 servings ½ cup cooked 1 cup fresh
Fruit group	2 servings ¼ cup ½ fresh	4 servings ½ cup 1 fresh
Fats and oils group	as needed ½ tbsp. oil ½ pat of butter	as needed 1 tbsp. oil 1 pat of butter

Encourage your child to eat what the rest of the family eats. You do not want to be forced to become a short-order cook. Abigail says, "I had a brother who was a fussy eater, and my mother catered to him day and night. But I didn't want to be a kitchen slave to my own kids, cooking special meals for each one. I tell my children, 'This is what we're having for dinner tonight. You can eat what you want, but I'm not preparing any special orders.'"

Now that your child is older, don't make the mistake of offering only one food at a time; if your child doesn't like it, there's no alternative. Instead, include a variety of foods at each meal, so that your child can pick and choose. For example, if you have an unpopular meat such as liver, try to have a favorite vegetable or starch, like corn. And always include bread and milk with each meal.

National dietary surveys show that children ages 6 to 11 often lack certain nutrients[6]. Here are the nutrients to watch for and some foods that can boost your child's intake of these nutrients (for additional sources, see Table 2-1 and Table 2-2):

- Vitamin A, found in cantaloupe, peaches, carrots, spinach, fish, eggs, and dairy foods.
- Vitamin E, found in whole grains, wheat germ, spinach, corn oil, soybean oil, and safflower oil.
- Vitamin C, found in oranges, strawberries, broccoli, and peppers.
- Vitamin B_6, found in bananas, brown rice, oats, peanuts, and whole wheat.
- Calcium, found in dairy foods, various green vegetables, salmon, sardines, and tofu.
- Iron, found in red meat, spinach, beans, raisins, and wheat cereal.
- Magnesium, found in bananas, avocados, beans, potatoes, oatmeal, peanuts, milk, and yogurt.
- Zinc, found in beans, whole grains, nuts, red meat, turkey, eggs, and yogurt.

Pay attention to your youngster's intake of calcium, needed to build strong teeth and bones: 500 mg per day at ages 1 to 3, and 800 mg per day at ages 4 to 8. Make milk at mealtimes the rule. Also take advantage of calcium-enriched foods. Light n' Lively cottage cheese and Kraft Singles American cheese slices have twice as much calcium as their regular cheese counterparts, and also provide protein, phosphorus, and vitamins A and B_{12}. Calcium-fortified orange juice, with 300 to 450 milligrams of calcium per 6-ounce serving is another smart choice. For more information, see another of my books: *The Complete Guide to Building and Maintaining the Healthiest Bones.*

THE LOWFAT/HIGH-FIBER MISTAKE

The food choices that are healthiest for adults are not necessarily the healthiest for young children. For instance, a lowfat/high-fiber diet has been recommended for adults as a means of weight control—yet unfortunately, this has become ingrained as the standard for everyone. Young children need foods with good fats. In early childhood, a lowfat/high-fiber diet is a prescription for malnutrition during the last critical period for metabolic programming, when many organs and body systems are completing their final stages of development. Without foods rich in fats, a young child cannot get enough calories or the critical essential fatty acids that come only from fats. This can impair a child's visual and neurological growth. The problem with excess fiber is that it fills a child up too quickly, leaving no room in a tiny tummy for other nutritious foods that are also vital to positive metabolic programming.

So please, do not be too quick to switch from whole milk to skim, to push peas instead of peanut butter, or to offer tofu in place of hamburgers. If you yourself are on a reducing diet, do not put your child on the diet, too. The American Academy of Pediatrics recommends that a minimum of 20 percent of calories in your child's diet (and a maximum of 30 percent) should come from fat, with no more than 10 percent of calories coming from saturated fat[7].

To determine in grams how much fat your child should be getting every day, add five to his or her age—for instance, a three-year-old needs about 8 grams of fat daily, while an eight-year-old needs about 13 grams. Here are examples of how to meet those needs:

- From age 1 to 3, a child's need for fats can be met with 8 ounces of milk, 2 ounces of meat, and ½ pat of butter.
- From age 4 to 8, a child's need for fats can be met with 18 ounces of milk, 6 ounces of meat, and 1 pat of butter.

The same equation applies to dietary fiber. While adults need 25 to 30 grams of fiber daily, a child's fiber intake (in grams) should roughly equal his or her age plus five. For instance:

- From age 1 to 3, a child's need for fiber can be met with two slices of bread, one and a half cups of fresh vegetables, and one fresh fruit.
- From age 4 to 8, a child's need for fiber can be met with one and a half cups of cereal, two slices of bread, one cup of pasta or rice, a salad, and two fresh fruits.

If you're concerned about a strong family history of heart disease or high cholesterol, speak to your pediatrician about having your child's cholesterol tested. In some cases, a special diet may be advisable.

THE TOP 25 FOOD ALL-STARS

The Top 25 Food All-Stars listed in Chapter 2 are just as important for your growing child as they were for you when you were pregnant, because each provides a concentrated dose of good nutrition. Your child may not immediately like all of them, of course. Simply continue to offer these foods in a low-pressure way, showing your child that you enjoy them, and eventually he or she will probably come to like most of them, too.

The recipes at the end of the book are rated according to the nutrient content per serving, as well as the number of All-Star foods included as ingredients. As a quick review, here are the Top 25 Food All-Stars:

• Yogurt	• Tofu	• Sweet potatoes, yams
• Milk	• Beans, peas,	• Tomatoes
• Cheese	lentils, chickpeas	• Apples
• Tuna, salmon	• Nuts	• Avocados
• Shellfish	• Asparagus	• Cherries
• Eggs	• Broccoli	• Oranges
• Lean beef	• Cabbage	• Oatmeal
• Lean pork	• Pumpkin	• Wheat germ
• Lean poultry	• Spinach	

Smart Snacking

Because children need to eat more than three times a day, snacks provide an excellent opportunity to fit more of the Top 25 Food All-Stars into your child's diet. For instance, one of the healthiest snacks you can give your child is a plate of cut-up raw vegetables with hummus or ricotta cheese for dipping, or fruit slices with yogurt or cottage cheese on the side. Try dried fruits such as raisins, prunes, dates, dried apple chips, or dried peaches, too. These types of snacks provide needed nutrients and calories without spoiling a child's appetite for dinner.

Marin, a mother of four, says, "I used to throw away apples and pears that had gone bad because my kids forgot they were in the kitchen. Then one day I sliced up some apples to salvage the parts that were still edible, and I brought the plate into the playroom. Ten minutes later my kids were asking for more! Now I buy all kinds of fruits and vegetables to cut into slices. I even bought an inexpensive hand-held slicer that makes ridges, like ruffled potato chips—but with zucchini and carrots instead of chips, snack time is so much healthier."

Fast-Food Strategies

Unfortunately, the Top 25 Food All-Stars are not often found at the fast-food restaurants kids love. Nor do most fast foods contain the good fats that children need. When you do buy fast food, improve the overall nutritional quality with these simple additions and changes:

- Order vegetables (onions, mushrooms, green peppers) on pizza.
- Ask that fast-food sandwiches and burgers be served without mayonnaise or cream-based sauces.
- Bring along fresh fruit and raw vegetables, or order a side salad.
- Order chili instead of a hamburger.
- Buy your child a baked potato instead of french fries.
- Order milk instead of soda for your child's beverage.

SAFETY TIPS TO REMEMBER

To reduce the risk of choking, make sure your child sits down for his snack. Do not offer popcorn or hard candies to any child under age four. For toddlers and preschoolers, food should be moist and tender; otherwise, it must be cut into small pieces (for instance, grapes, hot dogs, raw carrots, and nuts).

Follow the same food-safety measures you took when pregnant in preparing food for your child.

- Avoid unripened cheeses, which carry a risk of *Listeria* food poisoning.
- Avoid foods containing raw eggs (Caesar salad dressing, unpasteurized eggnog, raw cookie dough). Thoroughly cook eggs and egg-containing foods (scrambled eggs, French toast) to reduce the risk of *Salmonella* poisoning.
- Practice sanitary handling of raw meats. Do not serve undercooked beef, pork, or poultry, as these may be sources of *Trichinosis*, *Salmonella*, and *Campylobacter jejuni*.
- Check your water supply for lead content. Never allow your child to drink from ceramic mugs that may contain a lead glaze.

To reduce the risks of illness due to pesticides and bacteria from soil, clean all produce thoroughly before serving it. This goes for home-grown and organically grown produce, too; although these may not have the pesticides of regular produce, they are still grown in soil. Here are guidelines to follow:

- Wash produce in water. Or use a produce wash made from baking soda and citric acid, which helps to remove soil, wax, and pesticides; be sure to rinse thoroughly.
- Also use a produce brush to remove dirt and residue from the surfaces and crevices of fruits and vegetables.
- Discard the outer leaves of leafy vegetables such as lettuce and cabbage.

- Scrub the outside of melons with water or a produce wash; rinse thoroughly before cutting.
- Cut vegetables on a clean surface or board—not one that was just used for raw meat. Be sure to use a clean knife.
- Store produce on a shelf or drawer above raw meat in the refrigerator; otherwise the raw meat juices may drip on them and cause contamination. For added safety, seal raw meat in a plastic zipper bag before placing in the refrigerator.
- Keep your refrigerator produce drawer clean and sanitized.
- Peel apples, peaches, pears, carrots, and cucumbers. The skins of these fruits and vegetables are more likely to contain higher levels of pesticides, and your child can get plenty of fiber from other sources.

Think, too, about the caffeine in your child's diet. Even though he or she does not drink your coffee, your child may be consuming a significant amount of caffeine. Young children get about half their caffeine from carbonated beverages and half from cocoa and chocolate products, including ready-to-eat chocolate cereals[8]. By strictly limiting your child's consumption of these foods and beverages, you not only avoid the caffeine, but also a lot of unnecessary sugar.

Finally, remember that medications and vitamin or mineral supplements may look like candy to a young child, and even when only a few are eaten, the consequences can be tragic. For instance, iron supplements are the most common cause of pediatric poisoning deaths in the United States[9]. Be sure to keep all prescription and over-the-counter medications and supplements up high and locked away, well beyond your youngster's reach. Children are by nature curious individuals, busy exploring the environment around them. It's your job to make that environment safe so your child can learn and grow.

Obesity in Children:
A Growing Problem

Youngsters in the United States are getting fatter, and doing so at ever-younger ages. Nowadays, one out of every five children and adolescents in this country is overweight[10,11,12,13]. In children, *overweight* is defined as being above the eighty-fifth percentile of weight-for-height (according to the growth charts at the end of this chapter). Grown-ups are getting fatter, too: 63 percent of men and 55 percent of women aged 25 and older are now overweight (defined as a body mass index, or BMI, between 25 and 29.9) or obese (BMI of 30 or greater)[14,15].

This is a very disturbing trend, because obesity is a significant risk factor for diabetes, heart disease, and some forms of cancer[16,17]. In fact, heart disease and cancer are the leading causes of death in the United States—not just among the elderly or even the middle-aged, but among all men and women age 25 and older (see Table 9-1). What's more, the American Heart Association recently concluded that non-insulin-dependent diabetes is as great a risk factor for heart disease and stroke as smoking.

As the science of metabolic programming is now proving, a tendency to develop these diseases can lie dormant for years until triggered by obesity or some other negative factor later in life[18,19,20]. The risk is particularly high among individuals whose growth before birth was less than optimal. For instance, recent studies have shown the following:

- Men in the lowest third of ponderal index at birth (a measure for newborns that's similar to BMI) and the highest third of body mass in childhood had a fourfold increased risk of death from coronary heart disease[21,22].
- The prevalence of the insulin resistance syndrome was 25 percent for individuals whose birthweights were in the lowest third and whose current BMIs were in the highest third. By compari-

TABLE 9-4. LEADING CAUSES OF DEATH BY AGE AND GENDER, UNITED STATES, 1998
(Bold values are the top three causes of death within the age- and gender-specific category.)

MALES

	Ages 1–4		Ages 5–14		Ages 15–24		Ages 25–44		Ages 45–64		Ages 65+	
	Rank	Rate*	Rank	Rate	Rank	Rate	Rank	Rate	Rank	Rate	Rank	Rate
ALL CAUSES		37.6		23.4		119.3		208.8		836.9		5,582.4
Heart Disease	5	1.5	6	1.0	5	3.5	**2**	**28.5**	**2**	**253.2**	**1**	**1,906.1**
Malignant Neoplasms	4	2.4	**2**	**2.9**	4	5.4	4	23.4	**1**	**255.3**	**2**	**1,407.2**
Cerebrovascular Disease			9	0.2	8	0.6	8	4.1	4	30.6	**3**	**356.5**
Chronic Pulmonary Disease	9	0.4	7	0.4	7	0.8			7	24.3	4	347.8
Pneumonia & Influenza	6	0.9	8	0.3	9	0.6	10	2.7	9	13.0	5	252.1
Diabetes Mellitus							9	3.6	6	25.8	6	146.9
Accidents	**1**	**14.9**	**1**	**10.4**	**1**	**51.9**	**1**	**48.9**	**3**	**46.8**	7	113.9
Renal Disease											8	74.2
Septicemia	7	0.7									9	54.1
Alzheimer's Disease											10	48.7
Congenital Anomalies	**2**	**3.7**	5	1.0	6	1.3						
Homicide	**3**	**2.9**	**3**	**1.3**	**2**	**24.8**	6	15.0				
Perinatal Conditions	8	0.5										
Meningitis	10	0.4										
Suicide			4	1.2	**3**	**18.5**	**3**	**23.5**	8	22.4		
Benign Neoplasms			10	0.2	10	0.5						
HIV Infection							5	15.7	10	12.1		
Chronic Liver Disease & Cirrhosis							7	6.5	5	29.0		

*Rates per 100,000 population.

FEMALES

	Ages 1–4		Ages 5–14		Ages 15–24		Ages 25–44		Ages 45–64		Ages 65+	
	Rank	Rate*	Rank	Rate	Rank	Rate	Rank	Rate	Rank	Rate	Rank	Rate
ALL CAUSES		31.4		16.2		43.5		107.4		501.9		4754.9
Heart Disease	5	1.3	5	0.7	5	2.1	3	11.9	2	101.5	1	1,658.4
Malignant Neoplasms	4	2.4	2	2.3	3	3.7	1	28.1	1	209.9	2	912.7
Cerebrovascular Disease	9	0.4	10	0.2	9	0.5	7	3.9	3	23.3	3	438.2
Chronic Pulmonary Disease			7	0.3					4	21.2	4	240.2
Pneumonia & Influenza	6	1.0	8	0.3	7	0.6	10	1.9	8	8.2	5	233.6
Diabetes Mellitus					10	0.4	9	2.4	5	20.1	6	139.1
Accidents	1	10.5	1	6.1	1	19.1	2	16.5	6	18.0	7	83.2
Alzheimer's Disease											8	76.7
Renal Disease									10	5.2	9	59.9
Septicemia	8	0.5									10	56.1
Congenital Anomalies	2	3.7	4	0.9	6	1.1						
Homicide	3	2.4	3	1.1	2	4.3	6	4.6				
Perinatal Conditions	7	0.5										
Benign Neoplasms	10	0.3	9	0.2								
Suicide			6	0.4	4	3.3	4	6.0	9	6.4		
HIV Infection					8	0.6	5	5.1				
Chronic Liver Disease & Cirrhosis							8	2.9	7	10.1		

*Rates per 100,000 population.

Adapted from Murphy SL. Deaths: Final Data, 1998. National Vital Statistics Reports 2000; Vol. 48, No. 11.

son, the prevalence of insulin resistance syndrome was 0 percent for individuals whose birthweights were in the highest third and whose current BMIs were in the lowest third.

- Research suggests that poor growth before birth, particularly late in pregnancy when the liver is growing rapidly, may be related to elevated fibrinogen levels—a known risk factor for cardiovascular disease—in adult life[23,24]. Fibrinogen levels are even higher among individuals who were overweight during childhood[25].

What makes all of this a major concern for you as a parent is the fact that an overweight youngster is more likely to become an overweight adult[26]. The risk increases with the child's age: four out of ten obese seven-year-olds become obese adults, whereas eight out of ten obese adolescents continue to be obese as adults[27,28].

The risk is highest among children whose parents are also obese[29]. In other words, while your son or daughter may have inherited your beautiful eyes or winning smile, you also may have passed on your genetic predisposition to gain body fat—and therefore to develop chronic disease.

This is why it's so important that your youngster—particularly if he or she was undernourished before birth—not become overweight during childhood. However, I do not recommend that you put your child on a weight-loss diet. This can actually do more harm than good. A far better strategy is to help your child to stop gaining weight and allow his or her height to catch up to weight. To achieve this, your child needs to do three things:

- Follow the dietary guidelines in this chapter, taking smaller portions of high-calorie, high-fat foods like macaroni and cheese, and extra helpings of fresh fruits and vegetables.
- Get an appropriate amount of rest.
- Exercise regularly.

This last point—regular exercise—cannot be emphasized too strongly. Studies show that, although dietary patterns have remained fairly stable among children over the past several decades, physical activity has declined. The American Academy of Pediatrics' Committee on Sports Medicine and Fitness concludes that a low level of physical activity is the primary factor contributing to the development of obesity among children[30]. In other words, the main problem is not that today's kids eat too much—it's that they exercise too little.

Achieving and maintaining an ideal weight-for-height and overall physical fitness during childhood is key to preventing many chronic diseases. Studies show that body fat during childhood is linked to high blood cholesterol levels[31]. But exercise reduces the likelihood that this tendency will be triggered, even when there's a genetic predisposition to accumulate excess body fat[32]. Furthermore, moderate physical activity benefits the immune system. For instance, one recent study showed that a program of regular walking cut the number of respiratory infections in its participants in half[33].

How can you keep your child from being a junior couch potato? The very best way is by modeling good exercise habits yourself. If you need extra motivation, remember that an estimated 250,000 deaths in the United States each year (12 percent of total deaths) are attributable to a lack of regular exercise[34,35], yet one-third or more of all adults have no leisure-time physical activity. This proportion increases with age, is higher among women than among men, and is more common in winter months. Regular physical activity reduces your risk of diabetes, colon cancer, hypertension, osteoporosis, depression, and obesity, to name just a few.

The President's Council on Physical Fitness and Sports recommends a minimum of 30 minutes a day of physical activity for students in kindergarten through twelfth grade[36]. Right now, the most important step you can take to assure your child's positive metabolic programming—and to protect your own health—is to make a commitment to do some daily physical activity together. So turn off the TV and take your youngster outside. Ride your bicycles together, go for a walk, or play a good old-fashioned game of tag. Be sure family vacations include active time, too. Skiing, swimming, canoeing, hiking, biking, and tennis not only make for a fun family getaway, but they also promote your child's lifelong love of sports.

Adolescent Growth and Development

The growth patterns of boys and girls begin to differ as they approach the growth spurt of adolescence. Generally, boys grow the most between the ages of 12 to 16, adding as much as twelve inches in height and fifty to sixty pounds in weight. For the most part, boys reach their adult height by age 20, although some do grow another inch or so in their twenties. Young men continue to put on weight, mostly from added muscle, through their early thirties.

For girls, the adolescent growth spurt occurs earlier, typically between the ages of 10 and 14. During this time, girls add about ten inches in height and forty to fifty pounds in weight. Thereafter, growth in height slows significantly, and any additional weight comes primarily from body fat.

In general, children who were born heavy or large for their gestational age tend to remain taller than average with the onset of puberty. Conversely, those born light or short for gestational age usually remain shorter than average[37,38]. Children whose growth before birth was less than optimal also tend to have less muscle and more fat, as compared to children of the same weight who were well grown at birth[39,40].

This additional fat tends to be stored in the trunk and abdominal areas—a pattern that is strongly associated with an increase in blood pressure, high cholesterol, and the risks of diabetes and coronary heart disease[41,42,43,44]. The tendency to put on fat centrally is stronger in girls than in boys, particularly when weight gain is excessive during late adolescence or when a teenager smokes[45,46,47].

AGE AT PUBERTY: WHY IT MATTERS
Less-than-optimal growth before birth can also affect your child's age at puberty. Scientists suspect that both early puberty and delayed puberty among boys have some negative health effects, though it is unclear exactly what those consequences may be. Among girls, however, the adverse effects of early puberty and of delayed puberty are well documented.

The primary health issue for adolescent girls is menarche, the start of regular monthly menstrual cycles. Body weight and adequate body fat in the right combination trigger specific hormonal changes; these in turn initiate regular menstrual periods[48]. Some studies suggest that girls must attain a minimum of 17 percent body fat for menarche to occur, and must maintain at least 22 percent body fat in order to have regular menstrual cycles[49]. While the exact thresholds may vary from individual to individual (and also may be influenced by factors such as physical activity and stress), it does appear that lower-than-normal levels of body fat or weight can adversely affect menarche and menstrual cycles. (See Table 9-5.)

Girls who are short at birth, either symmetrically small (indicating slowed growth from the first trimester onward) or short but of normal birthweight (indicating slowed growth during the third trimester) tend to experience earlier menarche, perhaps brought on by their higher percentage of body fat. They are also likely to undergo earlier menopause[50,51]. Both of these occurrences have important health implications.

A girl who starts menstruating before age 12 tends to put on fat

TABLE 9-5. IDEAL WEIGHT-FOR-HEIGHT (BMI 19.8–26.0) AND
HIP MEASUREMENTS ASSOCIATED WITH 22–26% BODY FAT

Height	Weight Range (lb)	Hip Measurement
4'10''	95–125	30–32.5''
4'11''	98–129	31–33.5''
5'	102–134	31.5–34''
5'1''	105–138	32–34.5''
5'2''	109–143	32.5–35''
5'3''	112–147	33.5–36''
5'4''	116–152	34–36.5''
5'5''	120–157	34.5–37''
5'6''	123–162	35.5–38''
5'7''	127–167	36–38.5''
5'8''	131–172	36.5–39.5''
5'9''	135–177	37.5–40''
5'10''	139–182	38–40.5''
5'11''	143–187	38.5–41''
6'	145–193	39.5–42''

in the trunk and abdominal areas, which increases her risk for various chronic diseases, as discussed above. Early menarche also is associated with a higher incidence of breast cancer[52,53].

Early menopause means a woman has fewer years in which to bear children. She also has less time to build bone mass before age-related bone loss begins, and she is quicker to lose the protective effects of estrogen on the heart.

Other girls may experience a delay in menarche, meaning regular menstrual periods do not begin until age 14 or later. This may be due to low body fat, vigorous physical activity, or other disturbances of the normal hormonal balance. Delayed menarche raises the risk of poor bone health, both immediate and in the long run. That's because adolescence is a crucial period for rapid bone growth, when a girl should acquire as much as 37 percent of the bone mass she will carry into adulthood. When this growth is compromised, she is more likely to suffer stress fractures during the reproductive years. The risk rises as bone density drops after menopause. In fact, studies show that bone fractures occur three times more often among menopausal and postmenopausal women who experienced delayed menarche[54,55,56,57,58].

Your Adolescent's Nutritional Requirements

The nutritional needs of boys and girls are the same during early childhood. But as adolescence approaches, boys' and girls' dietary requirements diverge. Preteen and teenage boys need more calories than do girls (with a proportional increase in certain nutrients), while girls require more iron (see Table 9-6). By the time they reach the middle teen years, both boys and girls have the same nutritional requirements as adults, and should follow the adult recommendations for getting fewer than 30 percent of calories from fat, with less than 10 percent of calories coming from saturated fat, and no more than 300 mg of cholesterol per day.

NUTRIENTS TODAY'S TEENS LACK

What teenagers need to eat, unfortunately, is often the opposite of what they actually do eat. This means that, during the time when growth is most rapid and metabolic programming is in its final phase, many teenagers have diets deficient in an array of vital nutrients. Specifically, national dietary surveys show that children ages 12 to 19 tend to lack the same nutrients as their younger counterparts—vitamins A, E, C, B_6, and the minerals calcium, magnesium, zinc, and iron (as discussed earlier in this chapter)—in addition to the following:

TABLE 9-6. DIETARY REQUIREMENTS DURING LATE CHILDHOOD AND ADOLESCENCE

	MALES		FEMALES	
	9 to 13 years	14 to 18 years	9 to 13 years	14 to 18 years
Calories	2,000–2,500	2,500–3,000	2,000–2,200	2,200
Protein	28–45 g	45–59 g	28–46 g	44–46 g
Vitamin A	700–1,000 µg RE	1,000 µg RE	700–800 µg RE	800 µg RE
Vitamin B$_6$	1.0 mg	1.3 mg	1.0 mg	1.2 mg
Vitamin B$_{12}$	1.8 µg	2.4 µg	1.8 µg	2.4 µg
Vitamin C	45 mg	75 mg	45 mg	65 mg
Vitamin D	5 µg	5 µg	5 µg	5 µg
Vitamin E	11 mg	15 mg	11 mg	15 mg
Thiamin	0.9 mg	1.2 mg	0.9 mg	1.0 mg
Riboflavin	0.9 mg	1.3 mg	0.9 mg	1.0 mg
Niacin	12 mg	16 mg	12 mg	14 mg
Folate	300 µg	400 µg	300 µg	400 µg
Pantothenic Acid	4 mg	5 mg	4 mg	5 mg
Biotin	20 µg	25 µg	20 µg	25 µg
Choline	375 mg	550 mg	375 mg	400 mg
Calcium	1,300 mg	1,300 mg	1,250 mg	1,250 mg
Fluoride	2 mg	3 mg	2 mg	3 mg
Iodine	120–150 µg	150 µg	120–150 µg	150 µg
Iron	10–12 mg	12 mg	10–15 mg	15 mg
Phosphorus	460 mg	500 mg	460 mg	500 mg
Magnesium	240 mg	410 mg	240 mg	360 mg
Selenium	40 µg	55 µg	40 µg	55 µg
Zinc	10–15 mg	15 mg	10–12 mg	12 mg

Recommended Dietary Allowances (RDAs) and Dietary Reference Intakes (DRIs) from the Food and Nutrition Board of the National Academy of Sciences, 2000.

- thiamin, found in oranges, peas, beans, wheat germ, pasta, oatmeal, cereals, breads, beef, and pork
- riboflavin, found in various green vegetables, cereals, poultry, fish, and dairy foods
- folic acid, found in various green vegetables, oranges, beans, cereals, and beef liver
- vitamin B_{12}, found in seafood, milk, yogurt, pork, and beef liver

In recent times teenagers have doubled or tripled their consumption of carbonated beverages and cut their intake of milk by more than 40 percent. According to national dietary surveys conducted by the U.S. Department of Agriculture, 75 percent of teenage boys drink an average of 34 ounces of soda—that's nearly three 12-ounce cans—and only 16 ounces of milk daily. Among teenage girls, 66 percent drink 23 ounces of soda—almost two full 12-ounce cans—and a scant 12 ounces of milk daily. These habits leave today's teenagers woefully lacking in the calcium they need to protect their teeth and bones. Point of fact: Research shows a strong link between consumption of carbonated beverages and bone fractures among teenage girls, particularly those who are physically active[59]. To add more calcium to your child's diet, try these hints.

- Serve calcium-fortified orange juice (+300–450 mg per 6 oz).
- Try salmon burgers instead of hamburgers (+180 mg per 3 oz).
- Use evaporated nonfat milk in creamed soups (+600 mg per 8 oz).
- Add firm tofu to stir-fry dishes (+260 mg per ½ cup).
- Serve three-bean salad as a vegetable side dish (+120 mg per cup).
- Substitute calcium-fortified milk for regular milk (+200 mg per 8 oz).
- Change from ice cream to frozen yogurt (+350 mg per ½ cup).

Unlike younger children, for whom fiber intake should be more limited, teenagers do need plenty of fiber. Because of its insulin-lowering effects, a fiber-rich diet may reduce the risks for both obesity and cardiovascular disease[60]. As discussed in Chapter 2, fiber content is one of the factors affecting a food's glycemic index (a measure of the rate at which carbohydrates enter the bloodstream). Fiber helps the body maintain a stable level of blood sugar. Here are some strategies for adding more fiber to your teenager's diet:

- Double the fiber by substituting whole fruit for more processed versions (apples instead of applesauce, oranges instead of orange juice).
- Replacing white bread with whole wheat increases the fiber twofold.
- Add wheat germ to yogurt (+2 g per 2 tablespoons).
- Substitute Ry-Krisp or Crispbread for regular crackers (+3 g per cracker).
- Substitute peanut butter for butter on breakfast toast (+2 g per 2 tablespoons).
- Add cashews to stir-fried meals (+1.7 g per 1 oz).
- Serve baked beans instead of rice or mashed potatoes (+7 g per ½ cup).

Breakfast: The Meal That Matters Most
Many teenagers skip breakfast, particularly girls who are dieting. Yet breakfast offers an important boost in terms of blood sugar levels, with carbohydrates supplying quick energy while proteins and fats provide staying power until lunch. Breakfast improves brainpower, too. Studies show that children who eat breakfast concentrate better, have higher test scores, and demonstrate improved social abilities.

If your teen complains that mornings are too rushed for breakfast, get ready the night before by putting out a bowl, spoon, cereal box, and a piece of fruit. That way, all your child has to do in the morning is pour the milk. Breakfast on the run can also be nutritious if you pack a brown bag with a few portable foods such as yogurt, string cheese, little cheese rounds, snack-sized cottage cheese containers, hardboiled eggs, fresh or dried fruit, boxed juices, whole-wheat crackers, homemade muffins, granola bars, or individual boxes of ready-to-eat cereal. If your teenager's school serves breakfast, you can supplement the cafeteria fare with any of the foods mentioned above, as well as fiber-rich microwavable instant oatmeal.

Lunch: Beating the Cafeteria Blues
Regulations passed in 1995 require that school lunches meet the Dietary Guidelines for Americans, including no more than 30 percent of calories from fat and less than 10 percent of calories from saturated fat. Also, school meals must now provide one-third of the RDA for protein, vitamins A and C, iron, calcium, and calories.

The problem is that many youngsters don't like what is offered at school. In fact, studies document that school cafeteria food is thrown away 50 to 70 percent of the time! If your teenager complains about the taste of cafeteria food, suggest that he or she bring lunch from home instead. Keep your cupboards and refrigerator stocked with healthful lunchtime choices, paying attention to your teenager's personal preferences. Kids are much more likely to eat what they select themselves.

Dangerous Dieting
By the time your child reaches age 9, he or she should have a diet very similar to the one recommended in the Food Pyramid Guide—in other words, basically a normal adult diet. By following the Food Pyramid, your child should receive the appropriate calories and nutrients, in the proper balance, that are needed for good health.

Yet preteens and teens sometimes dread the additional pounds they gain as their bodies mature, and may lose perspective on body image. According to data from a recent national survey of adolescents aged 12 to 16, more than half of girls and one-fourth of boys who considered themselves overweight were actually of normal weight[61]. Particularly likely to feel pressured are girls who participate in ballet, gymnastics, and figure skating, sports in which a thin figure is highly prized.

For such youngsters, dieting seems to be the obvious answer. Yet dieting during adolescence can be dangerous, interfering with normal growth and perhaps delaying the onset of puberty[62]. Fad diets that severely limit calories or prohibit entire categories of food are especially harmful. If your child truly is overweight, ask a registered dietitian to suggest an appropriate regimen. Otherwise, simply encourage your teen to follow a healthful diet that provides the right number of calories.

- Boys ages 9 to 13 need 2,000 to 2,500 calories daily.
- Boys ages 14 to 18 need 2,500 to 3,000 calories daily.
- Girls ages 9 to 13 need 2,000 to 2,200 calories daily.
- Girls ages 14 to 18 need about 2,200 calories daily.

Combined with daily physical activity, this level of calorie consumption should allow your youngster to maintain his or her weight, gradually slimming down as height increases.

Teenagers and Exercise

Regular exercise is as beneficial for teenagers as it is for younger children and adults, and for all the same reasons. In addition, exercise in the teen years is critical to bone health. Physical activity now, when the growth rate of bones is naturally at its greatest level, is essential to the development of peak bone mass (the highest bone density achieved throughout life), as well as the maintenance of bone mass later in life[63,64,65,66,67,68,69,70].

During youth, the skeleton is most responsive to exercise because mineral is acquired on more bone surfaces. Indeed, active teens reach adulthood with 5 to 10 percent greater bone mass, which provides long-term protection against osteoporosis. What's more, teens who regularly participate in sports are more likely to be physically active later in life[71]. Taken together, the cumulative effect of regular exercise in adolescence and adulthood results in the best bone health at every age[72,73].

HOW MUCH IS TOO MUCH?
Unfortunately, some teens carry a commitment to exercise too far—and this can cause a variety of health problems. Vigorous training can adversely affect hormone levels (and therefore bone health) in adolescents. One study showed that, compared to male rowers and sedentary controls, male triathletes had lower serum testosterone levels[74]. Another study reported that, compared to sedentary male adolescents of the same age, cyclists who had trained an average of ten hours per week during the prior two years had significantly lower bone mass and bone density[75]. Heavy physical training also appears to depress the immune response[76].

In girls, extreme physical activity—particularly when combined with strict dieting to maintain a lean figure—can delay menarche, lead to irregular menstrual cycles, or even cause menstruation to cease altogether. This is indicative of a disturbance of normal hormonal levels, particularly estrogen, and can lead to rapid loss of bone mass. Possible consequences include the development of scoliosis (curvature of the spine) and stress fractures[77,78,79]. Even after physical activity is reduced, a calcium-rich diet is followed, and regular menstrual cycles return, the bone mass that was lost may never be completely recovered[80,81,82,83,84].

The solution, of course, is to encourage your teenager to exercise moderately, rather than at the extreme levels that can damage his or her short- and long-term health. If you are concerned about a possible "exercise addiction," discuss the matter with your child's pediatrician.

The Truth About Smoking

The teen years are the time when your child is most likely to first try cigarettes. The dangers are well known, and include increased risk for:

- lung cancer
- emphysema and bronchitis
- heart disease
- stroke
- cervical cancer
- impaired fertility

Smoking during adolescence also increases the tendency to deposit fat centrally[85]. This, as discussed earlier, is associated with an increased risk for cardiovascular disease and diabetes. Among individuals whose growth before birth was impaired, there is strong evidence that smoking is even more likely to trigger a dormant tendency to develop heart disease or cancer. This means that if your child was born early, small, or short, it's particularly important that he or she refrain from smoking.

How can you prevent your child from smoking? First, set a good example by not smoking yourself. Frankly discuss the long-term dangers. Also point out the immediate consequences that are closer to a teenager's heart—that smoking causes bad breath and wrinkles, that kissing a smoker is like licking an ashtray, that burn holes can ruin favorite garments, that cigarettes waste money that could otherwise be spent on clothes, movies, or a car. Jean, a mother of three, says, "I've promised to pay each of my children a thousand dollars on their twenty-first birthday if they have not developed a smoking habit. It's worth that much and more to protect their health—not to mention keeping my home smoke-free."

Looking Ahead

Metabolic programming is the basis for a revolutionary new approach to the prevention of chronic disease in the twenty-first century. It represents an enormous leap forward in the care of pregnant women, and in the preventive health practices for children and young adults.

As effective as it is, metabolic programming is not a lifetime guarantee—but neither is it a life sentence for your child. The healthy lifestyle that your child adopts as a teenager and adult contributes a great deal toward his or her long-term well-being.

Yet by following the recommendations in this book, you have given your child the best possible start toward a long and healthy life. You have taken the positive steps needed to bring into being, one baby at a time, the healthiest generation this world has ever seen.

CDC Growth Charts: United States

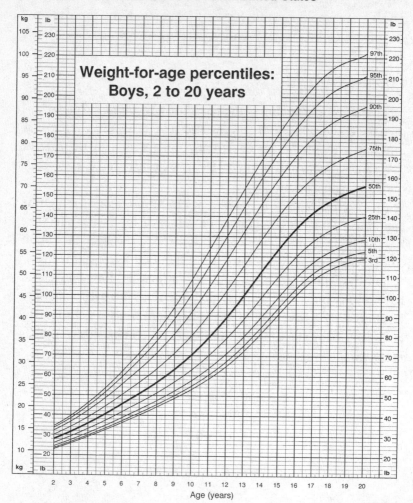

Weight-for-age percentiles: Boys, 2 to 20 years

Age (years)

SOURCE: Developed by the National Center for Health Statistics in collaboration with the National Center for Chronic Disease Prevention and Health Promotion (2000).

CDC Growth Charts: United States

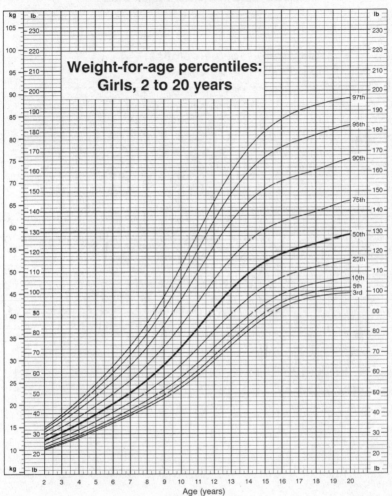

Weight-for-age percentiles:
Girls, 2 to 20 years

Age (years)

SOURCE: Developed by the National Center for Health Statistics in collaboration with the National Center for Chronic Disease Prevention and Health Promotion (2000).

CDC Growth Charts: United States

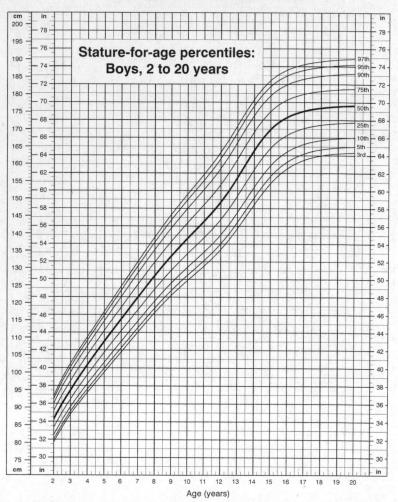

Stature-for-age percentiles:
Boys, 2 to 20 years

Age (years)

SOURCE: Developed by the National Center for Health Statistics in collaboration with
the National Center for Chronic Disease Prevention and Health Promotion (2000).

CDC Growth Charts: United States

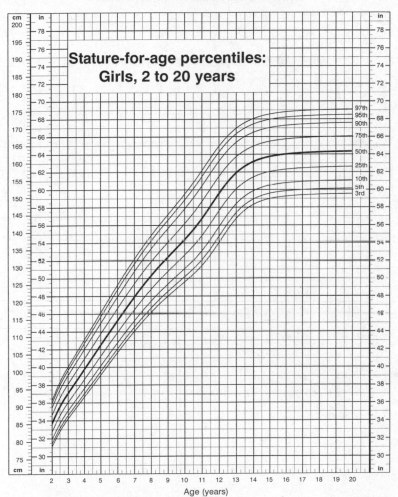

Stature-for-age percentiles:
Girls, 2 to 20 years

SOURCE: Developed by the National Center for Health Statistics in collaboration with
the National Center for Chronic Disease Prevention and Health Promotion (2000).

CDC Growth Charts: United States

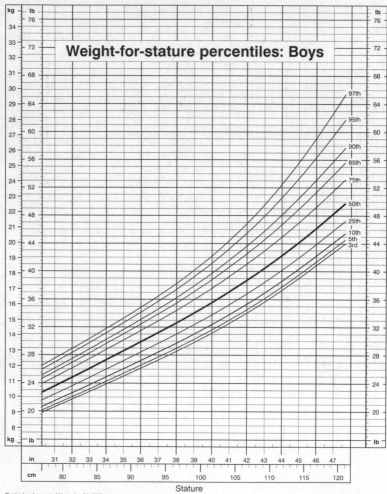

Weight-for-stature percentiles: Boys

Stature

Revised and corrected November 21, 2000.

SOURCE: Developed by the National Center for Health Statistics in collaboration with the National Center for Chronic Disease Prevention and Health Promotion (2000).

CDC Growth Charts: United States

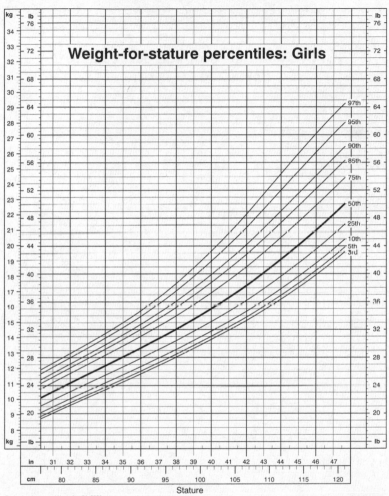

Weight-for-stature percentiles: Girls

Stature

Revised and corrected November 21, 2000.

SOURCE: Developed by the National Center for Health Statistics in collaboration with the National Center for Chronic Disease Prevention and Health Promotion (2000).

CDC Growth Charts: United States

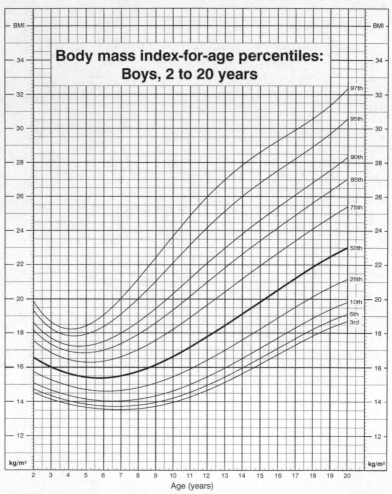

**Body mass index-for-age percentiles:
Boys, 2 to 20 years**

SOURCE: Developed by the National Center for Health Statistics in collaboration with
the National Center for Chronic Disease Prevention and Health Promotion (2000).

CDC Growth Charts: United States

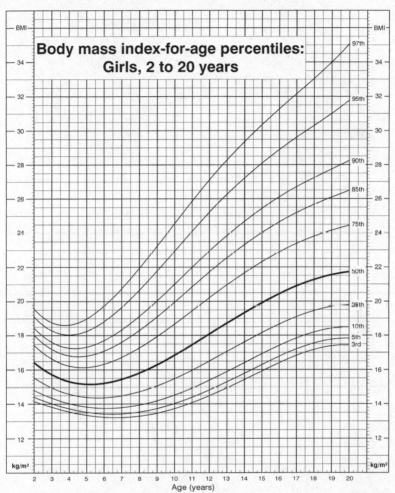

**Body mass index-for-age percentiles:
Girls, 2 to 20 years**

SOURCE: Developed by the National Center for Health Statistics in collaboration with
the National Center for Chronic Disease Prevention and Health Promotion (2000).

RECIPES

One of the most frequent questions I answer as a nutritionist caring for pregnant women is "What should I eat?" To help you put all the principles of good nutrition into practice, I have assembled sixty recipes in the following section, chosen primarily because of their nutritional content, but always keeping good taste in mind. The recipes have been analyzed using Nutritionist Five software, and list the nutrient composition per serving (calories, protein, carbohydrate, fat and saturated fat, calcium, iron, and fiber). In addition, each recipe is rated with stars for the number of nutrients present per serving at 20 percent or more of the RDAs for pregnancy, and with spoons for the number of Top 25 Food All-Stars included in the recipe. To help you look at these recipes in a different way, I have listed them below in terms of their star ratings (20 percent or more of certain nutrients per serving) for the B vitamins (including folic acid), the other vitamins (such as A, C, D), calcium and iron, the other minerals (such as phosphorus, magnesium, and selenium), and fiber.

	B Vitamins	Other Vitamins	Calcium and Iron	Other Minerals	Fiber
Beef					
Barbara's Meat Loaf	x			x	
Sunday Pot Roast	x	x		x	
Old-Time Beef Stew	x	x			x
Beef and Vegetable Lo Mein	x	x	x	x	x
Beef and Tomato Tacos				x	x
Shepherd's Pie	x	x	x	x	x
Southwest Salad	x			x	x
Baked Ziti with Meat Sauce	x	x		x	
Baked Eggplant Moussaka	x			x	
Poultry					
Chicken and Yam Stew	x	x		x	
Chicken and Dumplings	x	x		x	x
Chicken Cordon Bleu	x	x	x	x	
Cashew Chicken	x	x		x	
Chicken, Lentil, and Barley Soup	x	x		x	x
Bowties and Chicken with Peanut Sauce	x	x		x	
Turkey Breast with Cherries and Pecans	x			x	
Spinach-Stuffed Turkey Meat Loaf	x	x	x	x	
Asian Chicken Salad	x	x		x	

	B Vitamins	Other Vitamins	Calcium and Iron	Other Minerals	Fiber
Pork					
Hash Browns Supreme	x	x		x	
Baked Macaroni with Peas and Ham	x	x	x	x	
Cherry Glazed Pork Chops	x			x	
Hearty Bean Soup	x	x	x	x	x
Hearty Cassoulet	x	x	x	x	x
Sweet and Sour Pork	x	x		x	
Peanut Pork Chops	x	x		x	
Orange Pork Chops	x			x	
Seafood					
Creole Shrimp Bake	x	x		x	
Sylvia's Seafood Sauté	x	x		x	
Shrimp and Noodles with Peanut Sauce	x	x		x	
Fish Chowder	x	x		x	
Caesar Pasta Salad	x	x		x	
Salmon-Noodle Bake	x	x	x	x	
Tuna Casserole	x			x	
Salmon Fishcakes	x	x	x	x	
Shrimp Egg Foo Yung	x	x		x	
My Favorite Tuna Salad	x	x		x	
Sesame Tuna	x	x		x	
Seafood Bake	x		x	x	
Vegetarian					
Vegetarian Chili Lasagna	x	x		x	x
Mushroom-Spinach Bake	x	x	x	x	

	B Vitamins	Other Vitamins	Calcium and Iron	Other Minerals	Fiber
Spinach and Cheese Bake	x	x	x	x	
Vegetable Quiche	x	x	x	x	
Healthy Noodle Kugel	x			x	
Deluxe Green Beans			x		
Vegetable Tofu Stir-Fry	x	x		x	
Breads, Muffins, and Cakes					
Pumpkin Raisin Nut Muffins		x			
Date-Nut Bread	x			x	
Sunrise Muffins		x			
Daybreak Date Bread	x	x			
Very Berry Breakfast Cake		x			
Scottish Oat Scones					
Oatmeal Carrot-Cake Bread		x			
Quaker's Best Oatmeal Cookies					
Fruit Crisp Delight		x			x
Lemon Blueberry Muffins	x	x		x	
Lemon Yogurt Cookies					
Fruitful Morning Muesli	x	x		x	
Banana-Orange Oatmeal Muffins	x	x		x	
Wholesome Apple-Raisin Muffins	x	x		x	
Chewy Oatmeal Cookies					

Barbara's Meat Loaf

3   pounds extra-lean ground beef
1   cup prepared spaghetti sauce
1   (6-ounce) box seasoned croutons
4   egg whites, beaten
2   envelopes dry onion soup mix
2   (12-ounce) cans nonfat evaporated milk

1. Preheat oven to 375° F.
2. In large bowl combine beef, spaghetti sauce, croutons, egg whites, soup mix, and evaporated milk. Mix well. Divide mixture into two loaves and place into two 9 × 5 × 3-inch loaf pans.
3. Bake uncovered for 1½ hours; drain. Let stand 10 minutes before serving.

Makes 16 servings.

Nutrient Content Per Serving		★ Star Rating: 4		Spoon Rating: 4
Calories:	322 kcal	Vitamin B$_{12}$	86%	Beef
Protein:	22 g	Niacin	28%	Tomatoes
Carbohydrate:	18 g	Zinc	27%	Eggs
		Phosphorus	20%	Milk
Total Fat:	17 g			
Saturated Fat:	6.7 g			
Calcium:	167 mg			
Iron:	2.4 mg			
Dietary Fiber:	1.3 g			

Sunday Pot Roast

1   (3-pound) boneless beef roast, trimmed of fat
    Salt and pepper
1   (5-ounce) bottle prepared horseradish
1   cup water
8   small potatoes, peeled and halved
8   medium carrots, cut in 2-inch pieces
8   small onions, cut in half

1. Preheat oven to 325° F.
2. Place the roast on a rack in large roasting pan and season it with salt and pepper. Spread the horseradish over it. Add the water, cover with foil, and bake for 3 hours.
3. Uncover the roast and add the potatoes, carrots, and onions. Cook for an additional hour, or until meat and vegetables are tender.

Makes 10 servings.

Nutrient Content Per Serving		★ Star Rating: 11		⸡ Spoon Rating: 1
Calories:	462 kcal	Vitamin A	100%	Beef
Protein:	48 g	Vitamin C	26%	
Carbohydrate:	36 g	Iron	30%	
		Thiamin	31%	
Total Fat:	13 g	Niacin	41%	
Saturated Fat:	4.6 g	Vitamin B_6	42%	
		Vitamin B_{12}	100%	
Calcium:	69 mg	Phosphorus	39%	
Iron:	9.0 mg	Magnesium	24%	
		Zinc	83%	
Dietary Fiber:	4.1 g	Selenium	57%	

Old-Time Beef Stew

1	tablespoon olive oil
1½	pounds cubed lean stew beef, trimmed
2	medium onions, quartered
1	cup red wine
1	cup beef broth
4	medium sweet potatoes, cut into 1-inch cubes
4	stalks celery, cut into 1-inch pieces
6	carrots, cut into 1-inch pieces
½	teaspoon black pepper
1	tablespoon cornstarch
2	tablespoons cold water

1. In a large Dutch oven heat oil; add the beef and onions and sauté until the onions are tender.
2. Add the wine, broth, sweet potatoes, celery, carrots, and pepper.
3. Bring stew to a boil; reduce the heat and simmer, covered, for 45 minutes or until the beef is tender.
4. In a small cup, whisk together the cornstarch and cold water and gradually stir the mixture into the stew. Continue stirring until the sauce thickens. Cover and cook an additional 15 minutes, stirring occasionally.

Makes 8 servings.

Nutrient Content Per Serving		★ Star Rating: 5		🥄 Spoon Rating: 2
Calories:	258 kcal	Vitamin A	100%	Beef
Protein:	10 g	Vitamin C	51%	Sweet potatoes
Carbohydrate:	40 g	Vitamin B$_6$	27%	
		Vitamin B$_{12}$	40%	

Total Fat:	4.6 g	Fiber	22%
Saturated Fat:	1.6 g		
Calcium:	69 mg		
Iron:	2.0 mg		
Dietary Fiber:	6.5 g		

Beef and Vegetable
Lo Mein

1	pound beef flank steak
¼	cup barbecue sauce
¼	cup teriyaki sauce
2	tablespoons white wine vinegar
2	tablespoons peanut or sesame oil
1	(2-inch) piece fresh ginger, peeled and finely chopped
1	clove garlic, crushed
¼	cup water
2	ounces fresh snow peas
2	carrots, cut into ¼-inch rounds
1	(8-ounce) can pearl onions, drained
8	ounces of extra-firm tofu, cut into 1-inch cubes
4	cups uncooked fine egg noodles (about 8 ounces)
¼	cup chopped fresh cilantro

1. Cut beef across the grain into 2-inch strips. Place beef in shallow glass or plastic dish. In a small bowl, mix barbecue sauce, teriyaki sauce, and vinegar; pour half of the sauce mixture over the beef. Cover and marinate in the refrigerator for 2 to 4 hours. Refrigerate remaining sauce mixture.

2. In a large skillet or wok, heat oil over medium heat; add ginger and garlic and stir-fry for 2 minutes. Add marinated beef and stir-fry 4 to 6 minutes; add water and reserved sauce mixture, snow peas, carrots, pearl onions, and tofu; cover and cook 2 to 3 minutes or until vegetables are crisp-tender.

3. Cook noodles as directed on package and drain. Toss the noodles with ¼ cup of the sauce mixture from skillet. Divide the

noodles among 4 bowls and top with the beef and vegetables. Garnish with cilantro.

Makes 4 servings.

Nutrient Content Per Serving		★ Star Rating: 14		🥄 Spoon Rating: 3
Calories:	516 kcal	Phosphorus	38%	Beef
Protein:	39 g	Riboflavin	37%	Snow peas
Carbohydrate:	57 g	Folate	45%	Tofu
		Thiamin	60%	
Total Fat:	14 g	Vitamin B_6	33%	
Saturated Fat:	4 g	Niacin	62%	
		Magnesium	34%	
Calcium:	164 mg	Vitamin A	100%	
Iron:	6.3 mg	Vitamin C	24%	
		Vitamin B_{12}	100%	
Dietary Fiber:	4.1 g	Iron	21%	
		Fiber	39%	
		Selenium	98%	
		Zinc	56%	

Beef and Tomato Tacos

8   ounces lean ground beef
½   cup chopped onions
3   cloves garlic, minced
1   (16-ounce) can dark red kidney beans, undrained
6   taco shells
8   cups torn lettuce leaves (iceberg or romaine)
2   medium tomatoes, chopped
¾   cup shredded reduced-fat sharp cheddar cheese (about
    3 ounces)

1. In a medium skillet, brown the ground beef, and add the onions, and garlic. Drain off fat.
2. Stir in the kidney beans. Reduce heat, cover, and continue to cook for 10 minutes or until heated through.
3. To serve, divide the meat mixture among the taco shells. Top each with lettuce, tomatoes, and shredded cheese.

Makes 6 servings.

Nutrient Content Per Serving		★ Star Rating: 3		🥄 Spoon Rating: 4
Calories:	240 kcal	Phosphorus	21%	Beef
Protein:	18 g	Zinc	21%	Beans
Carbohydrate:	16 g	Fiber	22%	Tomatoes
				Cheese
Total Fat:	10 g			
Saturated Fat:	4.5 g			
Calcium:	131 mg			
Iron:	1.9 mg			
Dietary Fiber:	5.4 g			

Shepherd's Pie

2 teaspoons olive oil
12 ounces beef top round, cubed
2 cups chopped onions
1 cup sliced carrots
2 cups prepared beef gravy
1 (15-ounce) can kidney beans, drained and rinsed
1 cup canned tomatoes, undrained
3 cups cooked mashed potatoes

1. Preheat oven to 350°F.
2. In a large skillet, heat the oil over medium-high heat. Brown the beef and add the onions and carrots. Stir in the beef gravy and kidney beans; let simmer for 10 minutes. Add the tomatoes.
3. Pour the mixture into a large, deep casserole dish and top with mashed potatoes. Bake uncovered for 30 minutes or until potatoes brown slightly.

Makes 6 servings.

Nutrient Content Per Serving		★ Star Rating: 15		🥄 Spoon Rating: 3
Calories:	388 kcal	Potassium	30%	Beef
Protein:	30 g	Vitamin A	71%	Beans
Carbohydrate:	47 g	Vitamin C	30%	Tomatoes
		Iron	28%	
Total Fat:	9.5 g	Thiamin	23%	
Saturated Fat:	3 g	Niacin	29%	
		Vitamin B_6	39%	
Calcium:	83 mg	Folate	30%	
Iron:	5 mg	Vitamin B_{12}	25%	
		Phosphorus	34%	

Dietary Fiber:	10 g	Zinc	35%
		Copper	26%
		Manganese	46%
		Selenium	29%
		Fiber	40%

Southwest Salad

½   cup chopped onions
1   pound lean ground beef
1   teaspoon chili powder
2   teaspoons dried oregano
½   teaspoon ground cumin
1   cup canned red kidney beans, drained
1   (15-ounce) can chickpeas (garbanzo beans), drained
1   medium tomato, diced
2   cups shredded lettuce leaves
2   ounces shredded reduced-fat cheddar cheese

1. In a large skillet, cook onions and ground beef until the beef is no longer pink; drain off fat.
2. Add chili powder, oregano, and cumin to beef mixture; cook for 1 minute. Add the beans, chickpeas, and tomato. Stir gently to mix and heat thoroughly.
3. Combine lettuce and cheese in a large serving bowl; divide onto 6 plates. Top each with about 1 cup of beef mixture.

Makes 6 servings.

Nutrient Content Per Serving		★ Star Rating: 8		⸶ Spoon Rating: 5
Calories:	360 kcal	Riboflavin	20%	Beef
Protein:	22 g	Niacin	20%	Beans (2 kinds)
Carbohydrate:	25 g	Vitamin B_6	28%	Tomato
		Folate	20%	Cheese
Total Fat:	18 g	Vitamin B_{12}	31%	
Saturated Fat:	7 g	Phosphorus	27%	
		Zinc	29%	
Calcium:	109 mg	Fiber	25%	
Iron:	3 mg			
Dietary Fiber:	6.3 g			

Baked Ziti with Meat Sauce

8   ounces dried ziti
1   (16-ounce) can plum tomatoes, undrained
1   (3-ounce) can tomato paste
¼   cup red wine
½   teaspoon sugar
½   teaspoon crushed dried oregano
½   teaspoon crushed dried thyme
¼   teaspoon pepper
1   pound extra-lean ground beef
½   cup chopped onion
1   clove garlic, minced
1   cup shredded fat-free mozzarella cheese

1. Preheat oven to 375° F.
2. Cook pasta according to package directions; drain and set aside.
3. In a small bowl, mix tomatoes, tomato paste, wine, sugar, oregano, thyme, and pepper. Set aside.
4. In a large skillet, brown ground beef, onion, and garlic; drain off the fat. Stir in tomato mixture. Bring to a boil; reduce heat. Cover and simmer for 10 minutes. Stir in pasta.
5. Pour mixture into a 2-quart casserole dish and bake, uncovered, for 30 minutes. Sprinkle with mozzarella cheese. Bake 5 minutes more or until heated through.

Makes 6 servings.

Nutrient Content Per Serving

★ Star Rating: 6   🥄 Spoon Rating: 3

Calories:	309 kcal	Vitamin C	23%	Tomatoes
Protein:	27 g	Riboflavin	20%	Beef
Carbohydrate:	19 g	Niacin	27%	Cheese
		Vitamin B_{12}	77%	
Total Fat:	12 g	Zinc	30%	
Saturated Fat:	4.9 g	Selenium	22%	
Calcium:	134 mg			
Iron:	2.7 mg			
Dietary Fiber:	1.2 g			

Baked Eggplant
Moussaka

3   large eggplants (about 2 pounds each)
     Salt
     Olive oil (for coating eggplant) plus 1 tablespoon
4   cloves garlic, crushed
1   jumbo onion (about 1 pound), diced
2   pounds extra-lean ground beef
1   (8-ounce) can tomato paste
1   cup water
1   cup dry white wine
¼   teaspoon ground nutmeg
2   tablespoons chopped fresh parsley
     Pepper
1   (12-ounce) can evaporated skim milk
½   cup chicken broth
¼   cup flour
1   cup dry bread crumbs
¼   cup Parmesan cheese

1. Preheat oven to 425° F.
2. Peel and slice eggplant into ¼-inch slices; salt well and let stand for 1 hour. Rinse in cold water and drain.
3. Coat a large cookie sheet with olive oil and arrange the eggplant slices in a single layer. Brush eggplant slices with olive oil. Bake eggplant 15 minutes or until lightly browned. Remove eggplant from oven; turn oven temperature down to 350° F.
4. In a large skillet, heat 1 tablespoon olive oil and sauté garlic and onion until tender. Add ground beef and cook until browned. In a small bowl, combine the tomato paste and water; add

to skillet along with the wine, nutmeg, and parsley; season with salt and pepper to taste. Cover and let simmer for 5 to 7 minutes.

5. In a medium saucepan, combine the milk and chicken broth and heat. Gradually add the flour, whisking constantly until smooth. Cook over medium heat for about 10 minutes or until thickened, stirring frequently.

6. Sprinkle ⅓ of the bread crumbs on the bottom of a 13 × 9 × 2–inch baking dish. In layers, add ⅓ of the eggplant, ⅓ of the meat mixture, ⅓ of the white sauce, and ⅓ of the cheese. Repeat for 2 more layers with remaining eggplant, meat mixture, white sauce, and cheese.

7. Bake, uncovered, for 30 minutes or until golden brown. Cool slightly before serving.

Makes 10 servings.

Nutrient Content Per Serving		★ Star Rating: 6		Spoon Rating: 3
Calories:	350 kcal	Riboflavin	29%	Beef
Protein:	24 g	Niacin	36%	Tomatoes
Carbohydrate:	20 g	Vitamin B_6	20%	Cheese
		Vitamin B_{12}	91%	
Total Fat:	17 g	Phosphorus	24%	
Saturated Fat:	6.9 g	Zinc	30%	
Calcium:	200 mg			
Iron:	3.3 mg			
Dietary Fiber:	1.6 g			

Chicken and
Yam Stew

4	boneless, skinless chicken breasts
	Garlic salt
	Pepper
½	cup all-purpose flour
1	tablespoon olive or canola oil
2	cups cubed, peeled yams or sweet potatoes
1	cup chopped onion
1	cup chopped green pepper
¾	cup chicken broth
¾	cup apple cider

1. Rinse and pat dry chicken and cut into ½-inch pieces. Sprinkle with the garlic salt and pepper. Place the flour in a plastic bag; add the chicken, shaking until it is well coated with the flour.
2. In large skillet or Dutch oven over medium heat, heat the oil and brown the chicken on both sides just until golden brown. Remove chicken and set aside.
3. Add the yams or sweet potatoes, onion, and green pepper to the skillet; sauté until onion is tender. Stir in the chicken broth and apple cider. Add the browned chicken and bring to a boil. Reduce heat, cover, and simmer 25 to 30 minutes or until chicken is cooked through and the potatoes are tender.

Makes 4 servings.

**Nutrient Content
Per Serving**   ★ **Star Rating: 11**   ❘ **Spoon Rating: 2**

Calories:	494 kcal	Vitamin A	100%	Yams or sweet	
Protein:	60 g	Vitamin C	74%	potatoes	
Carbohydrate:	34 g	Vitamin E	25%	Chicken	
		Thiamin	20%		
Total Fat:	10 g	Riboflavin	28%		
Saturated Fat:	2 g	Niacin	100%		
		Vitamin B_6	44%		
Calcium:	58 mg	Vitamin B_{12}	22%		
Iron:	3.3 mg	Phosphorus	32%		
		Magnesium	22%		
Dietary Fiber:	3.7 g	Selenium	68%		

Chicken and
Dumplings

1	tablespoon safflower or olive oil
1	cup chopped onions
2	cups cooked, diced chicken
1	(14½-ounce) can diced tomatoes, undrained
2	(15-ounce) cans kidney beans, undrained
1½	cups reduced-fat all-purpose baking mix (like Bisquick)
½	cup cornmeal
⅔	cup skim milk
¼	cup sliced green onion
½	cup shredded 2% reduced-fat cheddar cheese

1. In a large skillet or Dutch oven, heat the oil and sauté the onions. Add the chicken, tomatoes, and beans; bring to a boil and reduce heat. Cover and simmer 5 minutes, stirring occasionally.
2. In a medium bowl, combine the baking mix, cornmeal, milk, and green onion. Mix until a soft dough forms, and drop by rounded spoonfuls onto the chicken mixture.
3. Cook uncovered, 10 minutes. Sprinkle with cheese. Cover and cook an additional few minutes until the cheese has melted.

Makes 6 servings.

Nutrient Content Per Serving		★ Star Rating: 5		🥄 Spoon Rating: 5
Calories:	374 kcal	Vitamin C	32%	Beans
Protein:	24 g	Riboflavin	20%	Chicken
Carbohydrate:	44 g	Niacin	26%	Tomatoes
		Selenium	20%	Milk
Total Fat:	12 g	Fiber	20%	Cheese

Saturated Fat:	4.3 g
Calcium:	166 mg
Iron:	2.3 mg
Dietary Fiber:	6.0 g

Chicken Cordon Bleu

⅓ cup diced onion
1 tablespoon chopped fresh parsley
2 tablespoons grated reduced-fat Parmesan cheese, divided
½ teaspoon pepper
½ teaspoon garlic powder
½ teaspoon paprika
4 boneless, skinless chicken breast halves, flattened to ⅛-inch thickness
4 (¾-ounce) slices reduced-fat Swiss cheese
4 thin slices cooked ham (about 2 ounces)
½ cup seasoned dry bread crumbs
⅓ cup all-purpose flour
2 eggs, beaten
2 tablespoons safflower oil
¾ cup chicken broth
¾ cup white wine
¼ cup sliced almonds (about 1 ounce)

1. In small bowl combine onion, parsley, 1 tablespoon Parmesan cheese, pepper, garlic powder, and paprika; mix well and set aside. On each chicken breast place one slice of Swiss cheese, one slice of ham, and one-fourth of the onion mixture. Roll up each chicken breast, folding ends to seal in the cheese and onion mixture, and fasten with toothpicks.
2. In a small bowl, combine the bread crumbs and the remaining tablespoon of Parmesan cheese. Roll each stuffed chicken breast in the flour, dip them into the beaten eggs, and then roll them in the bread crumb mixture.
3. In a large skillet, heat the oil over medium heat. Sauté the

chicken rolls, starting with seam side down, 7 to 10 minutes. Add the chicken broth and white wine; cover and continue cooking an additional 20 minutes. Top with sliced almonds and serve.

Makes 4 servings.

Nutrient Content Per Serving		★ Star Rating: 10		Spoon Rating: 6
Calories:	445 kcal	Vitamin B$_6$	30%	Chicken
Protein:	41 g	Vitamin B$_{12}$	54%	Cheese (2 kinds)
Carbohydrate:	21 g	Selenium	57%	Eggs
		Riboflavin	31%	Nuts
Total Fat:	21 g	Calcium	25%	Pork
Saturated Fat:	6 g	Phosphorus	39%	
		Niacin	66%	
Calcium:	300 mg	Vitamin A	20%	
Iron:	2.7 mg	Vitamin E	38%	
		Vitamin K	25%	
Dietary Fiber:	1.2 g			

Cashew Chicken

½   cup chicken broth
3   tablespoons oyster sauce
1½   tablespoons honey
1   tablespoon soy sauce
2   teaspoons white wine vinegar
1   tablespoon oil
1   pound skinned, boned chicken thighs, cut into bite-size pieces
1   cup chopped green onion, divided
½   cup sliced carrots
1   cup sliced mushrooms
1   cup snow peas
¼   cup canned pineapple chunks in juice, drained
⅓   cup cashews

1. In a small bowl, mix chicken broth, oyster sauce, honey, soy sauce, and vinegar.
2. In a large skillet or wok, heat oil over medium-high heat. Add chicken and cook until it turns white. Add the onion, carrots, mushrooms, snow peas, and pineapple and stir-fry for 2 to 3 minutes. Add the sauce, cover, and cook for an additional 2 to 3 minutes. Top with cashews and serve.

Makes 6 servings.

Nutrient Content Per Serving		★ Star Rating: 13		🥄 Spoon Rating: 3
Calories:	498 kcal	Vitamin A	56%	Snow peas
Protein:	28 g	Vitamin C	86%	Chicken
Carbohydrate:	62 g	Vitamin E	26%	Nuts

Total Fat:	15 g	Thiamin	41%
Saturated Fat:	2.9 g	Riboflavin	22%
		Niacin	52%
Calcium:	78 mg	Vitamin B_6	23%
Iron:	4.4 mg	Folate	32%
		Vitamin K	64%
Dietary Fiber:	3.1 g	Phosphorus	25%
		Magnesium	25%
		Selenium	49%
		Zinc	22%

Chicken Lentil and Barley Soup

½	cup dried lentils
2	tablespoons salted margarine or butter
1	cup chopped onion
1	clove garlic, minced
6	cups chicken broth
¼	teaspoon crushed dried oregano
¼	teaspoon crushed dried rosemary
¼	teaspoon pepper
1½	cups chopped cooked chicken
1½	cups sliced carrots
½	cup quick-cooking barley

1. Rinse and drain lentils, removing any debris.
2. Melt margarine or butter in a large saucepan or Dutch oven and sauté the onion and garlic until tender but not brown. Carefully stir in the chicken broth, oregano, rosemary, pepper, and lentils; bring to a boil. Reduce heat and simmer, covered, for 20 minutes.
3. Stir in the chicken, carrots, and uncooked barley. Simmer, covered, about 20 minutes more or until carrots and barley are just tender.

Makes 6 servings.

Nutrient Content Per Serving		★ Star Rating: 6		｜ Spoon Rating: 3
Calories:	260 kcal	Potassium	18%	Lentils
Protein:	21 g	Vitamin A	90%	Chicken

Carbohydrate:	25 g	Niacin	39%	Tomatoes
		Vitamin B_6	20%	
Total Fat:	8 g	Folate	22%	
Saturated Fat:	3.7 g	Phosphorus	26%	
		Fiber	30%	
Calcium:	41 mg			
Iron:	2.8 mg			
Dietary Fiber:	7.5 g			

Bowties and Chicken with Peanut Sauce

8   ounces dried enriched bowtie pasta
1   (14½-ounce) can chicken broth
2   tablespoons white wine
2   tablespoons oyster sauce
¼   teaspoon ground red pepper
¼   cup peanut butter
1   tablespoon canola oil
2   cloves garlic, minced
1   teaspoon grated fresh ginger
4   medium skinless, boneless chicken breasts (about
      12 ounces total), cut into 1-inch pieces
2   green onions, chopped
¼   cup crushed salted peanuts

1. Cook pasta according to package directions; drain.
2. In a medium bowl, mix chicken broth, wine, oyster sauce, red pepper, and peanut butter until smooth.
3. In a wok or large skillet, heat the oil; add the garlic and ginger and stir-fry for 2 to 3 minutes. Add the chicken and stir-fry about 3 minutes or until chicken is no longer pink. Remove the chicken and add the peanut butter mixture. Heat until thickened and bubbly. Add the chicken and cook for 2 minutes more.
4. In a large bowl, toss the pasta with the chicken and sauce and sprinkle each serving with green onions and peanuts.
Makes 4 servings.

Nutrient Content Per Serving

★ **Star Rating: 11**

🥄 **Spoon Rating: 2**

Calories:	525 kcal	Vitamin E	34%	Peanut Butter	
Protein:	41 g	Thiamin	46%	Chicken	
Carbohydrate:	52 g	Riboflavin	27%		
		Niacin	100%		
Total Fat:	16 g	Vitamin B_6	33%		
Saturated Fat:	3 g	Folate	40%		
		Vitamin B_{12}	20%		
Calcium:	49 mg	Vitamin K	32%		
Iron:	4 mg	Phosphorus	33%		
		Magnesium	29%		
Dietary Fiber:	3.1 g	Selenium	91%		

Turkey Breast with Cherries and Pecans

1   (3½-pound) turkey breast
1½   cups soft bread crumbs
½   cup dried cherries
¼   cup chopped toasted pecans
1   tablespoon salted margarine or butter, melted
2   tablespoons apple juice
¼   teaspoon crushed dried rosemary
1   tablespoon Dijon-style mustard
1   tablespoon olive oil

1. Preheat oven to 325° F.
2. Rinse the turkey and pat dry with paper towels. Cut a horizontal slit into thickest part of turkey breast to form a 5 × 4–inch pocket. Place the turkey in a shallow roasting pan.
3. In a medium bowl, combine bread crumbs, cherries, pecans, margarine or butter, apple juice, and rosemary. Spoon the stuffing into the pocket in the turkey. Fasten pocket opening securely with water-soaked wooden toothpicks or tie with heavy string.
4. In a small bowl, mix mustard and oil and brush the turkey with the mustard mixture. Insert a meat thermometer into the thickest part of the turkey breast.
5. Bake, uncovered, for 1½ to 2 hours, or until meat thermometer registers at least 180° F, basting with the mustard mixture during the last 15 minutes. Let stand for 15 minutes before slicing.
Makes 6 servings.

**Nutrient Content
Per Serving**   ★ Star Rating: 8   ❘ Spoon Rating: 3

Calories:	444 kcal	Riboflavin	23%	Turkey	
Protein:	67 g	Niacin	100%	Cherries	
Carbohydrate:	11 g	Vitamin B_6	72%	Nuts	
		Vitamin B_{12}	57%		
Total Fat:	13 g	Phosphorus	49%		
Saturated Fat:	2.7 g	Magnesium	31%		
		Zinc	25%		
Calcium:	52 mg	Selenium	100%		
Iron:	3.9 mg				
Dietary Fiber:	1.7 g				

Spinach-Stuffed Turkey Meat Loaf*

Nonstick cooking spray
1 cup coarsely chopped mushrooms
¼ cup chopped onion
1 (10-ounce) package frozen chopped spinach, thawed and drained
½ cup (2 ounces) shredded part-skim mozzarella cheese, divided
¼ cup grated Parmesan cheese
1 pound 99% lean ground turkey breast
¾ cup Quaker Oats (quick or old-fashioned, uncooked)
½ cup skim milk
1 egg white, lightly beaten
1 teaspoon Italian seasoning
½ teaspoon salt (optional)
¼ teaspoon pepper

1. Preheat oven to 375° F.
2. Lightly spray a 2-quart loaf pan with nonstick cooking spray. Sauté the mushrooms and onion over medium-low heat for 4 to 5 minutes or until the onion is tender. Remove from the heat; stir in the spinach, ¼ cup mozzarella cheese, and Parmesan cheese.
3. In a medium bowl, combine ground turkey, oats, milk, egg white, Italian seasoning, salt, and pepper. Mix lightly but thoroughly.
4. Spoon two-thirds of meat mixture lengthwise down center of the loaf pan; fill with spinach mixture. Top with remaining meat mixture, sealing edges to completely cover filling.

*From the Quaker Oats Company. Used with permission.

5. Bake 30 to 35 minutes or until the loaf reaches an internal temperature of 180° F when checked with a meat thermometer. Sprinkle with remaining cheese; return to oven 1 to 2 minutes or until cheese is melted. Let stand five minutes before slicing. Makes 6 servings.

Nutrient Content Per Serving		★ Star Rating: 9		🥄 Spoon Rating: 7
Calories:	204 kcal	Vitamin A	51%	Spinach
Protein:	27 g	Calcium	23%	Cheese (2 kinds)
Carbohydrate:	12 g	Riboflavin	22%	Turkey
		Niacin	32%	Oatmeal
Total Fat:	6 g	Vitamin B_6	24%	Milk
Saturated Fat:	2 g	Vitamin B_{12}	26%	Eggs
		Phosphorus	28%	
Calcium:	227 mg	Magnesium	29%	
Iron:	2.3 mg	Selenium	35%	
Dietary Fiber:	2.6 g			

Asian Chicken Salad

 2   green onions
1½   pounds chicken breasts, skinned, boned, and chopped
      into ½ × 2–inch strips
 ½   teaspoon peeled, minced fresh ginger
 1   teaspoon salt, divided
 ½   teaspoon pepper, divided
 4   tablespoons safflower oil, divided
 3   tablespoons lemon juice
 ½   teaspoon sugar
 3   cups finely shredded cabbage

1. Cut green tops of onions into 2-inch pieces, then cut each piece lengthwise into thin strips; set aside. Finely chop white part of onions. Combine chopped onion, chicken, ginger, ½ teaspoon salt, and ¼ teaspoon pepper.
2. Heat 2 tablespoons oil in a large skillet or wok and add the chicken mixture. Stir-fry just until chicken is opaque (about 3 minutes); remove chicken from wok; cool, cover, and chill.
3. Stir together lemon juice, sugar, and remaining 2 tablespoons oil, ½ teaspoon salt, and ¼ teaspoon pepper. Just before serving, mix together chilled chicken, lemon dressing, cabbage, and onion-top strips.

Makes 2 servings.

Nutrient Content Per Serving		★ Star Rating: 9		🥄 Spoon Rating: 2
Calories:	358 kcal	Vitamin C	26%	Chicken
Protein:	54 g	Vitamin E	34%	Cabbage
Carbohydrate:	4 g	Niacin	100%	

Total Fat:	13 g	Vitamin B$_6$	49%
Saturated Fat:	2 g	Vitamin B$_{12}$	26%
		Vitamin K	100%
Calcium:	56 mg	Phosphorus	34%
Iron:	2.2 mg	Magnesium	20%
		Selenium	72%
Dietary Fiber:	1.4 g		

Hash Browns Supreme

1	tablespoon safflower oil
2	cups frozen, shredded hash brown potatoes, thawed
¾	cup sliced green onion, divided
1½	cups seasoned croutons
2	eggs plus 6 whites, beaten
¾	cup diced reduced-fat, reduced-sodium ham
⅔	cup shredded reduced-fat cheddar cheese
¼	teaspoon coarsely ground pepper
	Salt to taste

1. In large skillet, heat oil; add the hash browns and ½ cup green onion. Fry about 8 to 10 minutes, or until potatoes are deep golden brown; stir occasionally.
2. Add the croutons, eggs, ham, cheese, and pepper. Cook until the eggs are set. Salt to taste. Garnish with the remaining green onions.

Makes 6 servings.

Nutrient Content Per Serving		★ Star Rating: 8		🥄 Spoon Rating: 3
Calories:	350 kcal	Vitamin B$_{12}$	20%	Eggs
Protein:	15 g	Niacin	21%	Ham
Carbohydrate:	30 g	Thiamin	20%	Cheese
		Riboflavin	24%	
Total Fat:	19 g	Selenium	28%	
Saturated Fat:	6 g	Phosphorus	20%	
		Vitamin E	26%	
Calcium:	75 mg	Vitamin K	46%	
Iron:	2.1 mg			
Dietary Fiber:	2.4 g			

Baked Macaroni
with Peas and Ham

2 tablespoons salted butter or margarine
2 tablespoons all-purpose flour
1 teaspoon dry mustard
2½ cups 1% milk
2 cups shredded cheddar cheese (about 8 ounces), divided
8 ounces dried enriched elbow macaroni
1 (10-ounce) package frozen sweet peas, thawed
8 ounces lean ham, cut into ½ × 1–inch strips
¼ cup seasoned bread crumbs

1. Preheat oven to 375° F.
2. In a large saucepan over medium heat, melt butter; whisk in the flour and mustard and mix well. Add the milk and stir until the sauce is smooth and slightly thickened. Add 1½ cups of cheese and heat until melted, stirring occasionally. Cover and remove from heat.
3. Meanwhile, cook the macaroni according to the package directions; drain. In a 2-quart casserole dish, combine the sauce with the macaroni, and add the peas and ham. Sprinkle with the remaining cheese and the bread crumbs.
4. Bake, uncovered, about 20 to 25 minutes, or until browned and bubbly.

Makes 8 servings.

**Nutrient Content
Per Serving**   ★ **Star Rating: 10**   ❘ **Spoon Rating: 4**

Calories:	341 kcal	Vitamin A	20%	Peas	
Protein:	21 g	Calcium	26%	Ham	
Carbohydrate:	35 g	Thiamin	47%	Milk	
		Riboflavin	30%	Cheese	
Total Fat:	12 g	Niacin	26%		
Saturated Fat:	7 g	Folate	25%		
		Vitamin B_{12}	34%		
Calcium:	315 mg	Phosphorus	31%		
Iron:	2.1 mg	Zinc	20%		
		Selenium	40%		
Dietary Fiber:	2.8 g				

Cherry Glazed Pork Chops

6   boneless pork chops, each ½ inch thick (about 1¼ pounds)
1   tablespoon safflower oil
1   teaspoon salt
½   cup maple syrup
½   cup hickory-flavored ketchup, or ¼ cup ketchup plus
     ¼ cup barbecue sauce
2   tablespoons lemon juice
2   teaspoons Worcestershire sauce
6   ounces dried cherries (or 12 ounces fresh, pitted)

1. In a large saucepan, brown pork chops in oil; sprinkle with salt; drain.
2. In a small bowl, combine the maple syrup, ketchup, lemon juice, and Worcestershire sauce. Pour half of this mixture over the pork chops. Cover and simmer for 30 minutes.
3. Add the remainder of the sauce and the cherries; simmer, covered, an additional 30 minutes.

Makes 6 servings.

Nutrient Content Per Serving		★ Star Rating: 8		Spoon Rating: 2
Calories:	374 kcal	Thiamin	69%	Pork
Protein:	28 g	Riboflavin	20%	Tomatoes
Carbohydrate:	31 g	Niacin	30%	
		Vitamin B$_6$	20%	
Total Fat:	15 g	Vitamin B$_{12}$	31%	

Saturated Fat:	4.7 g	Phosphorus	20%
		Zinc	22%
Calcium:	61 mg	Selenium	65%
Iron:	1.5 mg		
Dietary Fiber:	1.1 g		

Hearty Bean Soup

1	pound dried Great Northern beans
12	cups water, divided
2	cups beef broth
½	cup chopped onion
1	clove garlic, minced
2	cups cubed cooked ham
1	(14½-ounce) can Italian-style tomatoes, chopped
1	(10-ounce) package frozen chopped spinach, thawed and well drained
	Grated Parmesan cheese

1. Rinse beans and remove any sticks or debris. In a large saucepan or Dutch oven combine beans and 6 cups water; bring to a boil. Reduce heat and simmer for 2 minutes. Remove from heat. Cover and let stand 1 hour. Drain and rinse.
2. In the same pan, combine beans, 6 cups water, beef broth, onion, and garlic; bring to a boil. Reduce heat and simmer, covered, for 2 hours or until beans are tender. Add ham, tomatoes, and spinach and heat through. Sprinkle with Parmesan cheese.

Makes 6 servings.

Nutrient Content Per Serving		★ Star Rating: 10		🥄 Spoon Rating: 5
Calories:	227 kcal	Vitamin A	45%	Beans
Protein:	22 g	Vitamin C	27%	Tomatoes
Carbohydrate:	24 g	Calcium	24%	Spinach
		Iron	20%	Cheese
Total Fat:	4.8 g	Thiamin	40%	Ham
Saturated Fat:	2.1 g	Vitamin B_6	20%	
		Folate	34%	

Calcium:	236 mg	Phosphorus	32%
Iron:	3.5 mg	Magnesium	21%
		Fiber	31%
Dietary Fiber:	7.7 g		

Hearty Cassoulet

1   tablespoon canola oil
1   cup chopped onion
1   cup sliced carrots
8   ounces turkey, cubed
4   ounces ham, cubed
4   ounces pork sausage, cooked and diced
2   cups stewed tomatoes
1   cup chicken broth
2   (20-ounce) cans Great Northern beans, drained and rinsed
     Pepper to taste

1. Preheat oven to 350° F.
2. In a large saucepan or Dutch oven, heat oil over medium heat; add onions and carrots and sauté for 5 minutes.
3. Add turkey, ham, and sausage, and sauté another 5 minutes. Add tomatoes and chicken broth. Stir in beans and season with pepper.
4. Pour into a 2-quart casserole dish and bake uncovered for about 30 minutes or until bubbly.

Makes 8 servings.

Nutrient Content Per Serving		★ Star Rating: 11		🥄 Spoon Rating: 5
Calories:	340 kcal	Potassium	29%	Turkey
Protein:	28 g	Vitamin A	46%	Ham
Carbohydrate:	38 g	Vitamin C	20%	Pork
		Iron	25%	Tomatoes
Total Fat:	9 g	Thiamin	34%	Beans
Saturated Fat:	2.6 g	Niacin	27%	
		Vitamin B$_6$	23%	

Calcium:	138 mg	Folate	39%
Iron:	4.4 mg	Phosphorus	40%
		Magnesium	24%
Dietary Fiber:	11.4 g	Fiber	46%

Sweet and Sour Pork

Sauce

3	tablespoons cornstarch
¾	cup pineapple juice
¾	cup sugar
¾	cup vinegar
3	tablespoons soy sauce
3	tablespoons sherry
5	tablespoons ketchup

Marinade

½	teaspoon salt
½	teaspoon pepper
½	teaspoon sugar
2	tablespoons soy sauce
4	tablespoons sherry

1½	pounds lean pork, cut into 1-inch strips
2	tablespoons peanut oil
2	tablespoons grated fresh ginger
1	clove garlic, chopped
2	carrots, cut into ½-inch pieces
1	large onion, cut into ½-inch strips
4	green peppers, cut into 1-inch strips

1. In a small bowl, whisk together the cornstarch and pineapple juice. In a small saucepan, heat the ¾ cup sugar, vinegar, 3 tablespoons soy sauce, 3 tablespoons sherry, and ketchup. Bring to a boil and stir in the cornstarch mixture. Stir over low heat until thickened. Remove from heat.

2. In a medium bowl, combine the salt, pepper, ½ teaspoon sugar, 2 tablespoons soy sauce, and 4 tablespoons sherry. Add the pork, and marinate in the refrigerator for at least 20 minutes.

3. In a large skillet or wok, heat the oil and add the ginger and garlic. Stir-fry for 1 to 2 minutes. Add the marinated pork and cook until the pork is no longer pink. Add the carrots, onion, and peppers; stir-fry for 3 to 5 minutes, or until the vegetables are crisp-tender. Add the sweet and sour sauce and stir until heated through. Serve with hot rice.

Makes 6 servings.

Nutrient Content Per Serving		★ Star Rating: 9		ⵦ Spoon Rating: 1
Calories:	393 kcal	Vitamin A	100%	Pork
Protein:	26 g	Vitamin C	87%	
Carbohydrate:	45 g	Thiamin	79%	
		Riboflavin	22%	
Total Fat:	11 g	Niacin	31%	
Saturated Fat:	2.9 g	Vitamin B6	40%	
		Phosphorus	28%	
Calcium:	45 mg	Manganese	28%	
Iron:	2.9 mg	Selenium	67%	
Dietary Fiber:	2.0 g			

Peanut Pork Chops

4   boneless pork loin chops, ¾ inch thick (about 4 ounces each), well trimmed
3   tablespoons creamy peanut butter
1   tablespoon sugar
1   tablespoon soy sauce
⅛   teaspoon cayenne pepper
¾   cup water
1   tablespoon peanut oil
1   tablespoon peeled, minced fresh ginger
3   cloves garlic, crushed
4   medium green onions, cut into 1-inch diagonal slices

1. Broil pork chops until no longer pink inside, turning once. Transfer to a warm platter and cover with foil to keep warm.
2. Meanwhile, in a small bowl, whisk together peanut butter, sugar, soy sauce, cayenne pepper, and water until blended.
3. In a large skillet or wok, heat oil and add the ginger and garlic; sauté until browned; add the green onions. Add the peanut sauce and heat through.
4. Pour the peanut-onion mixture over the broiled pork chops.
Makes 4 servings.

Nutrient Content Per Serving		★ Star Rating: 10		🥄 Spoon Rating: 2
Calories:	349 kcal	Thiamin	88%	Pork
Protein:	38 g	Riboflavin	24%	Peanuts
Carbohydrate:	7 g	Niacin	47%	
		Vitamin B$_6$	27%	
Total Fat:	18 g	Vitamin B$_{12}$	38%	

Saturated Fat:	5.2 g	Vitamin K	50%
		Phosphorus	27%
Calcium:	51 mg	Magnesium	20%
Iron:	1.5 mg	Zinc	21%
		Selenium	83%
Dietary Fiber:	1.1 g		

Orange Pork Chops

½   cup fruit-only orange marmalade
¼   cup white balsamic vinegar
1   teaspoon salt
1   teaspoon coarse ground pepper
½   teaspoon ground cinnamon
½   teaspoon ground ginger
2   boneless pork loin chops, ¾ inch thick (about 4 ounces each)

1. In a small saucepan over low heat, cook marmalade and vinegar until marmalade is melted, stirring constantly.
2. In a small bowl, mix salt, pepper, cinnamon, and ginger. Rub spice mixture on both sides of each pork chop.
3. Broil pork chops, turning once or twice, until no longer pink inside. Brush them with marmalade glaze during last few minutes of cooking.

Makes 4 servings.

Nutrient Content Per Serving		★ Star Rating: 7		Spoon Rating: 1
Calories:	328 kcal	Thiamin	88%	Pork
Protein:	34 g	Riboflavin	22%	
Carbohydrate:	26 g	Niacin	37%	
		Vitamin B_6	24%	
Total Fat:	9 g	Vitamin B_{12}	38%	
Saturated Fat:	3.3 g	Phosphorus	23%	
		Selenium	82%	
Calcium:	52 mg			
Iron:	1.1 mg			
Dietary Fiber:	1.1 g			

Creole Shrimp Bake

1½ pounds cooked medium-size shrimp
1 cup chopped onion
1 cup chopped celery
½ cup chopped green pepper
1 (6-ounce) can tomato paste
1 tablespoon chopped fresh parsley
¼ teaspoon cayenne pepper
1 cup nonfat mayonnaise
6 ounces seasoned bread crumbs

1. Preheat the oven to 350° F.
2. In a large bowl, mix together the shrimp, onion, celery, green pepper, tomato paste, parsley, cayenne pepper, and mayonnaise.
3. Pour the mixture into a 2-quart casserole dish and sprinkle with bread crumbs.
4. Bake, uncovered, for 30 minutes.

Makes 6 servings.

Nutrient Content Per Serving		★ Star Rating: 9		Spoon Rating: 2
Calories:	320 kcal	Vitamin C	30%	Shrimp
Protein:	22 g	Vitamin D	35%	Tomatoes
Carbohydrate:	31 g	Vitamin E	33%	
		Niacin	21%	
Total Fat:	12 g	Vitamin B$_{12}$	46%	
Saturated Fat:	2.5 g	Vitamin K	100%	
		Phosphorus	20%	
Calcium:	79 mg	Magnesium	20%	
Iron:	3.3 mg	Selenium	62%	
Dietary Fiber:	2.3 g			

Sylvia's Seafood
Sauté

3   pounds frozen cooked shrimp
1   pound dried enriched small shell-shaped pasta
2   ounces salted butter or margarine
½   cup olive oil
6   cloves garlic, minced
½   cup dried parsley flakes
2   teaspoons crushed dried sweet basil
1   teaspoon dried oregano
2   (10½-ounce) cans minced clams, undrained
1   (26-ounce) jar marinara sauce
2   tablespoons grated Parmesan cheese

1. Thaw shrimp; drain and set aside.
2. Cook the pasta according to the package directions; drain and set aside.
3. In a large Dutch oven, heat the butter and oil, and sauté garlic; add the seasonings. Mix in the shrimp, pasta, clams, marinara sauce, and cheese.
4. Cover and simmer over low heat for 2 to 3 hours.
Makes 10 servings.

Nutrient Content Per Serving		★ Star Rating: 8		🥄 Spoon Rating: 4
Calories:	375 kcal	Vitamin A	23%	Shrimp
Protein:	36 g	Vitamin D	53%	Clams
Carbohydrate:	20 g	Vitamin E	23%	Cheese
		Niacin	30%	Tomatoes
Total Fat:	16 g	Vitamin B$_{12}$	76%	

Saturated Fat:	4.7 g	Phosphorus	27%
		Magnesium	20%
Calcium:	103 mg	Selenium	100%
Iron:	5.1 mg		
Dietary Fiber:	1.7 g		

Shrimp and Noodles with Peanut Sauce

8   ounces uncooked soba (buckwheat) noodles
1   tablespoon safflower oil
3   cloves garlic, finely chopped
1   tablespoon peeled and finely chopped fresh ginger
1   pound uncooked medium or large shrimp, peeled and deveined
2   cups shredded iceberg lettuce
1   (8-ounce) bottle of Thai peanut sauce

1. Cook noodles as directed on package; drain.
2. In a large skillet or wok, heat oil. Add garlic and ginger. Add shrimp and stir-fry about 3 minutes or until they are pink and firm. Remove from skillet.
3. In a large bowl, mix noodles, shrimp, lettuce, and peanut sauce.
Makes 6 servings.

Nutrient Content Per Serving		★ Star Rating: 6		🥄 Spoon Rating: 2
Calories:	305 kcal	Vitamin D	29%	Shrimp
Protein:	25 g	Niacin	20%	Peanut sauce
Carbohydrate:	37 g	Vitamin B_{12}	40%	
		Phosphorus	21%	
Total Fat:	7 g	Magnesium	21%	
Saturated Fat:	1.0 g	Selenium	45%	
Calcium:	66 mg			
Iron:	3.4 mg			
Dietary Fiber:	3.0 g			

Fish Chowder

½ pound fresh or frozen cod or haddock fillets
2 tablespoons salted margarine or butter
1 cup chopped onion
2 stalks celery, chopped
1 cup sliced fresh or canned mushrooms
1 clove garlic, minced
¼ cup all-purpose flour
¼ teaspoon crushed dried thyme
4 cups diced cooked potatoes
2 cups skim milk
3 cups bottled clam juice

1. Cut the fish into 1-inch pieces. In a large saucepan or Dutch oven, melt the margarine or butter and sauté the onion, celery, mushrooms, and garlic for 6 to 8 minutes or until vegetables are crisp-tender. Stir in flour and thyme. Add the potatoes, milk, and clam juice. Cook and stir until thickened and bubbly. Cook and stir for 1 minute more. Add the fish. Bring to a boil.
2. Reduce heat and simmer, uncovered, for 3 to 5 minutes more or until fish flakes easily with a fork.

Makes 6 servings.

Nutrient Content Per Serving		★ Star Rating: 8		🥄 Spoon Rating: 2
Calories:	274 kcal	Potassium	26%	Fish
Protein:	27 g	Vitamin C	23%	Milk
Carbohydrate:	29 g	Niacin	32%	
		Vitamin B_6	34%	
Total Fat:	5 g	Vitamin B_{12}	28%	

Saturated Fat:	2.8 g	Phosphorus	39%
		Magnesium	21%
Calcium:	167 mg	Selenium	57%
Iron:	2.1 mg		
Dietary Fiber:	2.7 g		

Caesar Pasta Salad

3   anchovy fillets, mashed
1   tablespoon chopped garlic
3   tablespoons olive oil
2   tablespoons lemon juice
2   cups cooked bowtie pasta
6   cups shredded romaine lettuce
2   cups plain croutons
¼   cup finely grated Parmesan cheese
    Coarsely ground black pepper to taste

1. In a blender container or food processor, combine anchovy fillets, garlic, oil, and lemon juice. Cover and process until smooth.
2. Toss cooked pasta with the anchovy mixture; add the shredded lettuce and croutons, and dish out onto individual plates. Top with cheese and sprinkle with pepper.

Makes 4 servings.

Nutrient Content Per Serving		★ Star Rating: 5		🥄 Spoon Rating: 2
Calories:	239 kcal	Vitamin A	23%	Fish
Protein:	9 g	Vitamin C	34%	Cheese
Carbohydrate:	26 g	Thiamin	25%	
		Folate	34%	
Total Fat:	11 g	Manganese	31%	
Saturated Fat:	2.6 g			
Calcium:	142 mg			
Iron:	2.5 mg			
Dietary Fiber:	3.6 g			

Salmon-Noodle Bake

12   ounces enriched egg noodles
1   cup whole milk
½   cup creamed cottage cheese
8   ounces canned salmon, drained
2   ounces shredded cheddar cheese
2   chopped scallions

1. Preheat the oven to 350° F.
2. Cook egg noodles according to package directions; drain.
3. Pour noodles into a bowl, add milk, cottage cheese, and salmon. Toss gently. Pour into a 2-quart casserole dish, sprinkle with cheddar cheese, and top with scallions.
4. Cover and bake for 20 minutes.
Makes 4 servings.

Nutrient Content Per Serving		★ Star Rating: 8		🥄 Spoon Rating: 4
Calories:	340 kcal	Calcium	24%	Salmon
Protein:	22 g	Vitamin D	25%	Milk
Carbohydrate:	43 g	Thiamin	22%	Cottage cheese
		Niacin	26%	Cheese
Total Fat:	8.5 g	Folate	29%	
Saturated Fat:	3.7 g	Vitamin B$_{12}$	36%	
		Magnesium	22%	
Calcium:	243 mg	Selenium	76%	
Iron:	2.9 mg			
Dietary Fiber:	1.9 g			

Tuna Casserole

12	ounces enriched egg noodles
14	ounces canned tuna, drained
12	ounces nonfat sour cream
¾	cup lowfat milk
1	cup drained canned green peas
1	cup pearl onions
1	cup drained canned mushrooms
¼	cup grated Parmesan cheese
2	tablespoons butter

1. Preheat oven to 350° F.
2. Cook egg noodles according to the package directions; drain. In a large bowl, mix noodles, tuna, sour cream, milk, peas, onions, and mushrooms. Pour into a 2-quart casserole dish.
3. Sprinkle the cheese over the top and dot with butter.
4. Bake uncovered for 35 to 40 minutes or until bubbly.

Makes 8 servings.

Nutrient Content Per Serving		★ Star Rating: 6		🥄 Spoon Rating: 4
Calories:	346 kcal	Thiamin	20%	Milk
Protein:	23 g	Niacin	26%	Cheese
Carbohydrate:	44 g	Folate	23%	Tuna
		Phosphorus	27%	Peas
Total Fat:	7.6 g	Manganese	20%	
Saturated Fat:	3.4 g	Selenium	86%	
Calcium:	126 mg			
Iron:	2.9 mg			
Dietary Fiber:	3.4 g			

Salmon Fishcakes

1	pound cooked salmon (fresh or canned)
2	large potatoes, cooked and mashed
¼	cup chopped onion
1	tablespoon finely chopped fresh parsley
1	tablespoon finely chopped green onions
1	stalk fresh celery, finely chopped
1	tablespoon lemon juice
	Flour
2	eggs, beaten
	Bread crumbs
2	tablespoons olive oil

1. Chop the salmon into small pieces. In a large bowl, mix the salmon, mashed potatoes, onion, parsley, green onions, celery, and lemon juice.
2. Form the mixture into 3-inch balls and flatten them slightly.
3. Roll the salmon cakes in flour, dip them in the beaten egg, and then roll in bread crumbs.
4. In a large skillet, heat the oil and brown the salmon cakes.

Makes 4 servings.

Nutrient Content Per Serving		★ **Star Rating: 9**		▮ **Spoon Rating: 2**
Calories:	296 kcal	Vitamin C	22%	Salmon
Protein:	22 g	Vitamin D	100%	Eggs
Carbohydrate:	22 g	Vitamin B$_6$	27%	
		Vitamin B$_{12}$	100%	
Total Fat:	13 g	Niacin	44%	

Saturated Fat:	3.1 g	Potassium	22%
		Calcium	24%
Calcium:	283 mg	Phosphorus	100%
Iron:	1.8 mg	Selenium	100%
Dietary Fiber:	2.7 g		

Shrimp Egg Foo Yung

2   tablespoons peanut oil
8   ounces fresh shrimp, cooked, deveined, peeled, and
    drained
2   green onions, chopped
2   ounces fresh bean sprouts
1   teaspoon salt
1   teaspoon pepper
3   eggs plus 6 egg whites, beaten with 6 tablespoons water

1. In a large skillet or wok, heat oil. Add shrimp, green onions, bean sprouts, and salt and pepper, and stir-fry until the vegetables are tender.
2. Add egg mixture. Brown on one side; turn by sliding onto a large, flat dish, then turning back onto pan. Brown other side and maybe serve with hot rice.

Makes 2 servings.

Nutrient Content Per Serving		★ Star Rating: 11		⸙ Spoon Rating: 2
Calories:	354 kcal	Vitamin A	26%	Shrimp
Protein:	44 g	Vitamin D	53%	Eggs
Carbohydrate:	5 g	Vitamin E	24%	
		Vitamin K	40%	
Total Fat:	16 g	Riboflavin	59%	
Saturated Fat:	3.8 g	Niacin	20%	
		Folate	20%	
Calcium:	120 mg	Vitamin B$_{12}$	100%	
Iron:	4.5 mg	Phosphorus	33%	
		Magnesium	23%	
Dietary Fiber:	3.6 g	Selenium	100%	

My Favorite
Tuna Salad

1 (6-ounce) can chunk-light tuna packed in water, drained
¼ cup finely chopped celery
1 tablespoon minced onion
3 tablespoons light mayonnaise
¼ teaspoon paprika

1. In a small bowl, combine all ingredients with a fork.
2. Serve immediately, or cover and refrigerate.
Makes 2 servings.

Nutrient Content Per Serving		★ Star Rating: 4		Spoon Rating: 1
Calories:	157 kcal	Vitamin E	20%	Tuna
Protein:	22 g	Niacin	67%	
Carbohydrate:	4 g	Vitamin B_{12}	100%	
		Selenium	100%	
Total Fat:	5 g			
Saturated Fat:	1 g			
Calcium:	15 mg			
Iron:	1.4 mg			
Dietary Fiber:	0.3 g			

Sesame Tuna

1   tuna steak (about 1 pound), chopped
2   tablespoons reduced-sodium soy sauce
1   teaspoon peeled, grated fresh ginger
¼   teaspoon coarsely ground black pepper
1   green onion, chopped
¼   cup plain dry bread crumbs
2   tablespoons sesame seeds
1   tablespoon peanut or olive oil

1. In a medium bowl, mix tuna with soy sauce, ginger, pepper, and green onion. Shape mixture into four patties.
2. In a medium bowl, mix bread crumbs and sesame seeds. Dip tuna patties into the bread crumb mixture, turning to coat both sides. In a large skillet, heat the oil and sauté the tuna patties over medium heat until browned on both sides.

Makes 4 servings.

Nutrient Content Per Serving		★ Star Rating: 9		🥄 Spoon Rating: 1
Calories:	222 kcal	Vitamin A	93%	Tuna
Protein:	29 g	Thiamin	24%	
Carbohydrate:	7 g	Riboflavin	21%	
		Niacin	63%	
Total Fat:	8 g	Vitamin B$_6$	26%	
Saturated Fat:	1.8 g	Vitamin B$_{12}$	100%	
		Phosphorus	28%	
Calcium:	73 mg	Magnesium	27%	
Iron:	2.5 mg	Selenium	66%	
Dietary Fiber:	0.9 g			

Seafood Bake

1   (9-inch) pastry shell
1   tablespoon butter or margarine
2   tablespoons minced onions
1   (3-ounce) can sliced mushrooms, drained and the liquid reserved
2   eggs plus 4 egg whites, beaten
¾   cup light cream
½   teaspoon salt
⅛   teaspoon crushed tarragon
¼   teaspoon marjoram
     Dash cayenne pepper
⅛   teaspoon black pepper
¼   pound cooked and flaked mild white fish or crab
½   cup shredded reduced-fat Swiss cheese
     Paprika for garnish

1. Preheat oven to 375° F (350° F if using a glass baking dish).
2. Partially bake pastry shell following package instructions and let cool.
3. In a medium saucepan melt the butter and sauté the onions until tender. Add all but 10 slices of mushrooms. Continue to sauté until heated through.
4. In a medium bowl, combine the eggs, light cream, mushroom liquid, salt, tarragon, marjoram, cayenne, and pepper. Fold in sautéed onions and mushrooms and flaked fish. Pour the mixture into the pastry shell and sprinkle with cheese.
5. Bake for 20 minutes; top with extra mushrooms, and bake an additional 15 minutes until puffed and a knife inserted near the

center comes out clean. Let stand for 5 minutes before cutting.
Garnish with paprika.
Makes 4 servings.

Nutrient Content Per Serving		★ Star Rating: 5		❘ Spoon Rating: 4
Calories:	250 kcal	Calcium	24%	Fish
Protein:	19 g	Riboflavin	28%	Eggs
Carbohydrate:	8 g	Vitamin B$_{12}$	100%	Milk
		Phosphorus	21%	Cheese
Total Fat:	15 g	Selenium	43%	
Saturated Fat:	6 g			
Calcium:	238 mg			
Iron:	1 mg			
Dietary Fiber:	0.6 g			

Vegetarian Chili Lasagna

1   tablespoon butter or margarine
1   tablespoon safflower or olive oil
½   cup chopped onion
½   cup chopped green bell pepper
1   stalk celery, chopped
1   medium clove garlic, crushed
2   (15-ounce) cans black beans, rinsed and drained
2   (15-ounce) cans tomato sauce
¼   cup chopped fresh cilantro
1   (12-ounce) package of 1% cottage cheese
2   (8-ounce) packages reduced-fat cream cheese (Neufchâtel), softened
¼   cup nonfat sour cream
9   dried lasagna noodles, cooked and drained

1. Preheat oven to 350° F. Grease a 3 × 9 × 2–inch baking dish with butter or margarine.
2. In a large skillet, heat oil and sauté onion, pepper, celery, and garlic; cook until the vegetables are tender.
3. Add the black beans, tomato sauce, and cilantro and heat through.
4. In a medium bowl, combine the cottage cheese, cream cheese, and sour cream.
5. Cover the bottom of the greased baking dish with 3 noodles. Top with one-third of the sauce and one-third of the cheese mixture. Repeat layers twice, ending with the cheese mixture.
6. Bake, uncovered, for 40 to 45 minutes. Remove from the oven and let stand 10 minutes.

Makes 8 servings.

**Nutrient Content
Per Serving** ★ **Star Rating: 11** ❘ **Spoon Rating: 3**

Calories:	355 kcal	Vitamin B$_{12}$	24%	Beans	
Protein:	22 g	Folate	53%	Cheese	
Carbohydrate:	52 g	Thiamin	29%	Tomatoes	
		Riboflavin	21%		
Total Fat:	7 g	Magnesium	37%		
Saturated Fat:	3.7 g	Phosphorus	27%		
		Selenium	23%		
Calcium:	122 mg	Vitamin A	29%		
Iron:	4.3 mg	Vitamin C	34%		
		Vitamin E	20%		
Dietary Fiber:	12 g	Fiber	50%		

Mushroom-Spinach Bake

2   (15-ounce) can sliced mushrooms, drained
1   (10-ounce) package frozen chopped spinach, thawed and drained
1   (15-ounce) carton part-skim ricotta cheese
¼   cup grated reduced-fat Parmesan cheese
½   teaspoon crushed dried basil
½   teaspoon crushed dried thyme
1½ cups skim or 1% milk
2   eggs plus 2 egg whites
¼   teaspoon ground nutmeg
¼   teaspoon pepper
    Butter or margarine
8   thin slices of whole wheat or sourdough bread, halved

1. In large bowl, mix the mushrooms and spinach; set aside. In a second medium-size bowl, combine ricotta and Parmesan cheese, basil, and thyme; set aside. In a third medium bowl whisk together milk, eggs, egg whites, nutmeg, and pepper.
2. Grease a 11 × 7 × 2–inch baking dish with butter or margarine. Arrange 8 half-slices of bread in the bottom of the dish. Top with the spinach mixture, then add the ricotta mixture. Arrange the remaining 8 half-slices on top. Pour the egg mixture slowly over the bread, using a spatula to press down on the bread until the egg mixture is absorbed. Cover and refrigerate 8 to 24 hours.
3. Preheat the oven to 350° F.
4. Bake for 50 to 60 minutes or until the eggs are set and the casserole is golden brown. Let stand 10 minutes before serving.

Makes 6 servings.

Nutrient Content Per Serving ★ **Star Rating: 10** | **Spoon Rating: 5**

Calories:	279 kcal	Vitamin B$_{12}$	32%	Spinach
Protein:	20 g	Vitamin A	66%	Cheese (2 kinds)
Carbohydrate:	28 g	Calcium	36%	Milk
		Riboflavin	41%	Eggs
Total Fat:	10 g	Folate	27%	
Saturated Fat:	5 g	Phosphorus	28%	
		Magnesium	22%	
Calcium:	430 mg	Niacin	20%	
Iron:	2.4 mg	Selenium	52%	
		Thiamin	20%	
Dietary Fiber:	2.7 g			

Spinach and Cheese Bake

1   1 tablespoon butter
8   slices of white enriched bread
2   tablespoons salted margarine or butter
1   cup chopped onion
2   (10-ounce) packages frozen chopped spinach, thawed and
    well drained
    Dash salt and pepper
1½ cups shredded nonfat Swiss cheese (about 6 ounces), divided
2   eggs plus 2 egg whites, beaten
2½ cups skim milk

1. Grease a 2-quart rectangular baking dish with butter. Cover the bottom of the dish with half of the bread slices, trimming them to fit.
2. In a medium saucepan over medium heat, melt the margarine or butter. Add the onion; sauté until tender. Stir in the spinach, add salt and pepper, and cook for 3 minutes more.
3. Spread the spinach mixture over the layer of bread in the baking dish. Sprinkle 1 cup of the Swiss cheese over the spinach and bread. Layer the remaining bread slices over the Swiss cheese layer.
4. In a medium bowl, stir together the eggs, egg whites, and milk and pour over the layers in the baking dish. Cover and refrigerate at least 1 hour.
5. Preheat the oven to 375° F. Remove the cover from the dish and sprinkle the remaining Swiss cheese over the top. Cover and bake for 45 minutes. Uncover and bake about 15 minutes more or until heated through. Let stand, covered, for 10 minutes before cutting into squares for serving.

Makes 4 servings.

**Nutrient Content
Per Serving**   ★ **Star Rating: 10**   ❗ **Spoon Rating: 4**

Calories:	320 kcal	Vitamin A	100%	Spinach
Protein:	20 g	Vitamin C	20%	Cheese
Carbohydrate:	27 g	Calcium	57%	Eggs
		Thiamin	21%	Milk
Total Fat:	15 g	Riboflavin	42%	
Saturated Fat:	8.4 g	Folate	47%	
		Phosphorus	39%	
Calcium:	570 mg	Magnesium	29%	
Iron:	4.8 mg	Manganese	53%	
		Selenium	30%	
Dietary Fiber:	3.5 g			

Vegetable Quiche

½ cup all-purpose flour
1 teaspoon baking powder
2 eggs plus 6 egg whites, beaten
1 (10-ounce) package frozen chopped spinach, thawed and well drained
2 tablespoons salted butter or margarine, melted
1 cup grated carrots
½ cup chopped onion
2 cups small-curd 1% cottage cheese
2 cups shredded reduced-fat cheddar cheese (about 8 ounces)
2 cups shredded Monterey Jack cheese (about 8 ounces)

1. Preheat oven to 400° F.
2. In a large bowl, stir the flour and baking powder into the eggs and egg whites. Stir in the spinach, melted butter or margarine, carrots, onion, cottage cheese, cheddar, and Monterey Jack.
3. Pour the mixture into a 3-quart rectangular baking dish. Bake for 15 minutes. Reduce the oven temperature to 350° F; bake for 25 to 30 minutes more or until the quiche is puffed and the center is set. Remove from the oven and let the quiche stand for 15 to 20 minutes before cutting it into squares.

Makes 8 servings.

Nutrient Content Per Serving		★ Star Rating: 7		🥄 Spoon Rating: 5
Calories:	340 kcal	Vitamin A	85%	Eggs
Protein:	27 g	Calcium	54%	Spinach
Carbohydrate:	12 g	Riboflavin	34%	Cheese (3 kinds)
		Folate	20%	

Total Fat:	19 g	Vitamin B_{12}	20%
Saturated Fat:	12 g	Phosphorus	45%
		Zinc	20%
Calcium:	536 mg		
Iron:	1.5 mg		
Dietary Fiber:	1.9 g		

Healthy Noodle Kugel

1   (10-ounce) package egg noodles
2   eggs plus 4 egg whites
¾   cup sugar plus 1½ teaspoons sugar, divided
1   teaspoon vanilla extract
2   (8-ounce) cartons nonfat sour cream
2   cups nonfat cottage cheese
1   cup skim milk
2   tablespoons salted butter or margarine
½   teaspoon ground cinnamon
3   ounces sliced almonds

1. Preheat the oven to 350° F.
2. Cook the noodles according to the package directions. Drain and set aside.
3. In a large mixing bowl, beat the eggs, egg whites, ¾ cup sugar, and vanilla. Add the sour cream, cottage cheese, and milk; mix well. Stir in the cooked and drained noodles.
4. In a 13 × 9 × 2–inch baking pan, melt the butter or margarine. Pour the noodle mixture into the baking pan.
5. In a small bowl, stir together the 1½ teaspoons sugar and the cinnamon. Sprinkle the mixture on top of the noodles, then dot with the sliced almonds.
6. Bake for 60 to 75 minutes or until a knife inserted near the center comes out clean. The top should be nicely browned. Cool slightly before slicing into squares.

Makes 12 servings.

**Nutrient Content
Per Serving**   ★ Star Rating: 3   ⎪ Spoon Rating: 4

Calories:	290 kcal	Riboflavin	24%	Eggs
Protein:	15 g	Phosphorus	20%	Cheese
Carbohydrate:	40 g	Selenium	30%	Milk
				Nuts

Total Fat: 7 g
Saturated Fat: 2 g

Calcium: 117 mg
Iron: 1.5 mg

Dietary Fiber: 1.5 g

Deluxe Green Beans

1	tablespoon butter
2	(10-ounce) packages frozen French-style green beans
¼	cup shredded reduced-fat Swiss cheese
2	tablespoons butter or margarine
2	tablespoons flour
¼	teaspoon salt
¼	teaspoon pepper
1½	cups 1% milk
½	cup chopped almonds

1. Preheat oven to 375° F. Grease a shallow 1½- to 2-quart rectangular baking dish with butter.
2. Cook the green beans in boiling water for 5 minutes and drain them.
3. Layer the green beans and cheese in the prepared baking dish.
4. In a medium saucepan, melt the butter or margarine. Stir in the flour, salt, and pepper, and add the milk. Cook, stirring, until thickened and bubbly.
5. Pour the sauce over the vegetable mixture, lifting the mixture gently with a fork so the sauce will penetrate. Do not stir.
6. Bake, uncovered, for 20 to 30 minutes or until bubbly and heated through.
7. Sprinkle the almonds over the casserole and serve.

Makes 8 servings.

Nutrient Content Per Serving

★ Star Rating: 1

❘ Spoon Rating: 4

Calories:	170 kcal	Calcium	20%	Beans
Protein:	7 g			Cheese
Carbohydrate:	13 g			Milk
				Nuts

Total Fat:	10 g
Saturated Fat:	4 g

Calcium:	185 mg
Iron:	1.2 mg

Dietary Fiber:	3.4 g

Vegetable Tofu
Stir-Fry

1   cup water
¼   cup white wine
2   tablespoons soy sauce
4   teaspoons cornstarch
½   teaspoon sugar
1   tablespoon peanut oil
1   teaspoon grated ginger
1   clove garlic, chopped
2   cups carrots, cut into ½-inch pieces
1   pound fresh asparagus, cut into 1-inch pieces, or
     1 (10-ounce) package frozen cut asparagus, thawed and well
     drained
2   green onions, cut into 1-inch pieces
1   (10½-ounce) package extra-firm tofu, cut into ½-inch cubes
½   cup chopped almonds

1. In a small bowl, whisk together water, wine, soy sauce, corn-starch, and sugar.
2. In a large skillet or wok, heat the oil and add the ginger and gar-lic. Stir-fry for 2 to 3 minutes. Add the carrots; stir-fry for 3 minutes. Add the asparagus and green onions; stir-fry about 1½ minutes more or until the asparagus is crisp-tender. Re-move the vegetables.
3. Add tofu to the skillet or wok. Stir-fry for 2 to 3 minutes or until lightly browned. Remove from wok. Stir the soy sauce mixture and add it to the skillet or wok. Cook, stirring, until thickened and bubbly. Add cooked vegetables and tofu. Stir all ingredients together to coat with sauce. Cover and cook about

1 minute more or until heated through. Stir in almonds. May serve over rice.

Makes 4 servings.

Nutrient Content Per Serving		★ Star Rating: 6		🥄 Spoon Rating: 3
Calories:	178 kcal	Vitamin A	100%	Asparagus
Protein:	10 g	Vitamin C	36%	Tofu
Carbohydrate:	13 g	Vitamin E	35%	Nuts
		Folate	24%	
Total Fat:	9 g	Vitamin K	92%	
Saturated Fat:	1.1 g	Magnesium	23%	
Calcium:	74 mg			
Iron:	2.1 mg			
Dietary Fiber:	3.8 g			

Pumpkin Raisin Nut Muffins

1	tablespoon butter
1	(16-ounce) package nut-bread mix
1	(16-ounce) can pumpkin
1	egg, beaten
1	tablespoon sugar
½	teaspoon ground cinnamon
½	teaspoon ground nutmeg
½	cup raisins
1	cup chopped walnuts

1. Preheat oven to 375° F. Grease the bottoms of a large muffin tin with butter (or use paper muffin cups).
2. In a large bowl, combine bread mix, pumpkin, egg, sugar, cinnamon, and nutmeg until just moistened. Stir in raisins and walnuts.
3. Spoon into prepared muffin tin, filling each cup ¾ full.
4. Bake 20 to 25 minutes or until wooden pick inserted in the center of a muffin comes out clean. Let cool on a wire rack for 5 minutes; remove from pans.

Makes 12 muffins.

Nutrient Content Per Serving		★ Star Rating: 1		🥄 Spoon Rating: 3
Calories:	222 kcal	Vitamin A	100%	Pumpkin
Protein:	5 g			Egg
				Nuts
Carbohydrate:	37 g			
Total Fat:	6 g			
Saturated Fat:	1 g			

Calcium:	40 mg
Iron:	1.9 mg
Dietary Fiber:	2.5 g

Date-Nut Bread

	Butter or margarine
½	cup sugar
3	tablespoons safflower oil
1	egg, beaten
1	teaspoon vanilla extract
2½	cups all-purpose flour
3½	teaspoons baking powder
½	teaspoon salt
1	cup snipped dates
1	cup chopped nuts

1. Preheat oven to 350° F. Grease a 9 × 5 × 3–inch loaf pan with butter or margarine.
2. In a large bowl, combine the sugar, oil, egg, and vanilla, stirring until just mixed.
3. In another large bowl, stir together the flour, baking powder, and salt. Add the flour mixture to the sugar mixture and mix well. Stir in the dates and nuts. Pour the batter into the prepared pan.
4. Bake for 45 to 50 minutes or until a wooden pick inserted near the center comes out clean.
5. Cool the bread for 10 minutes in the pan. Then remove the bread from the pan and cool thoroughly on a wire rack. Wrap and store the bread overnight.

Makes 1 loaf.

Nutrient Content Per Serving		★ Star Rating: 4		🥄 Spoon Rating: 3
Calories:	350 kcal	Thiamin	22%	Egg
Protein:	8 g	Riboflavin	20%	Milk

Carbohydrate:	50 g	Copper	20%	Nuts
		Magnesium	20%	
Total Fat:	9 g			
Saturated Fat:	1.5 g			
Calcium:	67 mg			
Iron:	2.3 mg			
Dietary Fiber:	2.5 g			

Sunrise Muffins

1	tablespoon butter
2	cups all-purpose flour
1	cup apple butter
2	teaspoons baking powder
2	teaspoons ground cinnamon
½	teaspoon baking soda
¼	teaspoon salt
2	cups finely shredded carrots (about 2 to 3 medium carrots)
½	cup raisins
½	cup chopped nuts
½	cup chopped dates
2	eggs plus 2 egg whites
½	cup safflower oil
½	cup molasses
1	teaspoon vanilla extract

1. Preheat oven to 350° F. Lightly grease eighteen 2½-inch muffin tins with butter or line them with paper baking cups.
2. In a large mixing bowl, stir together the flour, apple butter, baking powder, cinnamon, baking soda, and salt. Stir in the carrots, raisins, nuts, and dates.
3. In a separate bowl, stir together the eggs, egg whites, oil, molasses, and vanilla. Add the liquid ingredients all at once to the flour mixture and stir just until moistened.
4. Gently spoon the batter into the prepared muffin cups until each one is almost full.
5. Bake for about 30 minutes or until the top of a muffin springs back when lightly touched. Cool in the pan set on a wire rack

for 5 minutes. Remove the muffins from the pan and let them cool on the rack. Serve warm or at room temperature.

Makes 18 muffins.

Nutrient Content Per Serving		★ **Star Rating: 2**		❘ **Spoon Rating: 2**
Calories:	280 kcal	Vitamin A	36%	Eggs
Protein:	4 g	Vitamin E	20%	Nuts
Carbohydrate:	46 g			
Total Fat:	9 g			
Saturated Fat:	0.8 g			
Calcium:	87 mg			
Iron:	1.6 mg			
Dietary Fiber:	2.2 g			

Daybreak Date Bread *

1	tablespoon butter
2½	cups all-purpose flour
1	cup uncooked Quaker Oats (quick or old-fashioned)
½	cup sugar
2	teaspoons baking powder
½	teaspoon baking soda
½	teaspoon salt (optional)
¾	cup chopped dates or raisins
¾	cup orange juice
¾	cup mashed ripe banana (about 2 medium)
½	cup safflower or canola oil
2	eggs, lightly beaten
2	teaspoons grated orange peel
1	teaspoon vanilla extract

Glaze

½	cup powdered sugar
3–4	teaspoons orange juice
½	teaspoon grated orange peel

1. Preheat oven to 350° F. Grease and flour the bottom of a 9 × 5–inch loaf pan with butter.
2. In a large bowl, combine flour, oats, sugar, baking powder, baking soda, salt, and dates or raisins; mix well. In a separate medium bowl, combine the orange juice, banana, oil, eggs, orange peel, and vanilla. Add wet ingredients to dry ingredients and mix just until dry ingredients are moistened.
3. Pour into prepared pan. Bake 60 to 70 minutes or until wooden

*From the Quaker Oats Company. Used with permission.

pick inserted in center comes out clean. Cool 10 minutes in pan; remove to wire rack. Cool completely.

4. For the glaze, combine the powdered sugar, orange juice, and orange peel; mix until smooth. Drizzle over bread.

Makes 12 servings.

Nutrient Content Per Serving		★ **Star Rating: 2**		❘ **Spoon Rating: 3**
Calories:	306 kcal	Vitamin E	41%	Oatmeal
Protein:*	5 g	Thiamin	20%	Eggs
Carbohydrate:	49 g			Oranges
Total Fat:	11 g			
Saturated Fat:	1 g			
Calcium:	17 mg			
Iron:	1.8 mg			
Dietary Fiber:	2.4 g			

Very Berry
Breakfast Cake*

Streusel
½   cup uncooked Quaker Oats (quick or old-fashioned)
¼   cup sugar
2   tablespoons margarine
¼   teaspoon ground cinnamon

Coffee Cake
½   cup (1 stick) margarine or butter, softened
1   cup sugar
4   egg whites, lightly beaten
1   (8-ounce) carton fat-free sour cream
1   teaspoon vanilla extract
1½   cups all-purpose flour
¾   cup uncooked Quaker Oats (quick, old-fashioned)
2   teaspoons baking powder
½   teaspoon baking soda
⅓   cup raspberry preserves
¾   cup fresh or frozen blueberries

1. Preheat oven to 350° F. Grease a 9-inch square baking pan with butter.
2. In a medium bowl, combine the streusel ingredients—the oats, sugar, margarine, and cinnamon—and cream together with a fork. Set aside.
3. For the cake, in a large bowl, beat together the margarine and sugar until creamy. Add the egg whites, sour cream, and vanilla;

*From the Quaker Oats Company. Used with permission.

beat well. In a medium bowl, combine the flour, oats, baking powder, and baking soda and add to the batter. Mix just until dry ingredients are moistened.

4. Spread the batter in the prepared pan. Spoon the raspberry preserves over the top and swirl them through the batter with a knife. Sprinkle the blueberries evenly over the batter, and sprinkle the streusel mixture over the blueberries.

5. Bake 50 to 55 minutes or until a wooden pick inserted in the center comes out clean; serve warm. Store leftovers tightly covered.

Makes 12 servings.

Nutrient Content Per Serving		★ Star Rating: 1		⸕ Spoon Rating: 2
Calories:	293 kcal	Vitamin A	20%	Oatmeal
Protein:	5 g			Eggs
Carbohydrate:	42 g			
Total Fat:	12 g			
Saturated Fat:	6 g			
Calcium:	38 mg			
Iron:	1.3 mg			
Dietary Fiber:	1.4 g			

Scottish Oat Scones*

1½   cups all-purpose flour
1   cup uncooked Quaker Oats (quick or old-fashioned)
¼   cup sugar
1   tablespoon baking powder
¼   teaspoon salt (optional)
½   cup (1 stick) margarine or butter, chilled
½   cup currants
⅓   cup milk
1   egg, lightly beaten
1   tablespoon sugar
⅛   teaspoon ground cinnamon

1. Preheat oven to 400° F. Grease a cookie sheet.
2. In a large bowl, combine the flour, oats, sugar, baking powder, and salt; mix well. Cut in the margarine with a pastry knife or two knives until mixture resembles coarse crumbs. Stir in currants.
3. In a small bowl, combine the milk and egg; add to the dry ingredients and mix with a fork just until dry ingredients are moistened.
4. Turn out onto a lightly floured surface; knead gently 8 to 10 times. Roll or pat dough into an 8-inch circle about ½ inch thick. Combine sugar and cinnamon and sprinkle on the dough. Cut the dough into 10 wedges and place them on the prepared cookie sheet.
5. Bake 12 to 15 minutes or until lightly golden brown. Serve warm.

Makes 10 scones.

*From the Quaker Oats Company. Used with permission.

Variations: Substitute raisins, dried cherries, cranberries, blueberries, or other diced dried fruit for currants, if desired.

Nutrient Content Per Serving		★ Star Rating: 0	▮ Spoon Rating: 3
Calories:	245 kcal		Oatmeal
Protein:	4 g		Milk
Carbohydrate:	32 g		Egg
Total Fat:	11 g		
Saturated Fat:	6 g		
Calcium:	26 mg		
Iron:	1.5 mg		
Dietary Fiber:	1.8 g		

Oatmeal
Carrot-Cake Bread*

1	1 tablespoon butter
1	cup uncooked Quaker Oats (quick or old-fashioned)
½	cup skim milk
2½	cups all-purpose flour
1	cup firmly packed brown sugar
1	tablespoon baking powder
½	teaspoon baking soda
½	teaspoon ground cinnamon
¼	teaspoon salt (optional)
1½	cups shredded carrots (about 3 medium)
½	cup raisins
1	(8-ounce) can crushed pineapple in juice, undrained
2	egg whites
¼	cup vegetable oil
1	teaspoon vanilla extract

1. Preheat oven to 350° F. Grease the bottom of a 9 × 5–inch loaf pan with butter.
2. In a medium bowl, combine oats and milk; mix well. Set aside. In large bowl, combine flour, sugar, baking powder, baking soda, cinnamon, and salt; mix well. Stir in carrots and raisins.
3. In a large bowl, combine reserved oat mixture, pineapple (including juice), egg whites, vegetable oil, and vanilla; mix well. Add to dry ingredients; mix just until dry ingredients are moistened.
4. Pour into prepared pan. Bake 60 to 75 minutes or until wooden

*From the Quaker Oats Company. Used with permission.

pick inserted in center comes out clean and crust is golden. Cool 10 minutes on a wire rack, then remove from pan and let bread cool completely.

Makes 16 servings.

Nutrient Content Per Serving		Star Rating: 2		Spoon Rating: 3
Calories:	212 kcal	Vitamin A	38%	Oatmeal
Protein:	4 g	Vitamin E	20%	Eggs
Carbohydrate:	39 g			Milk
Total Fat:	5 g			
Saturated Fat:	0.6 g			
Calcium:	36 mg			
Iron:	1.7 mg			
Dietary Fiber:	1.6 g			

Quaker's Best Oatmeal Cookies*

1	cup (2 sticks) margarine, softened
¾	cup firmly packed brown sugar
½	cup granulated sugar
1	egg
1	teaspoon vanilla extract
1½	cups all-purpose flour
1	teaspoon baking soda
½	teaspoon salt (optional)
1	teaspoon ground cinnamon
¼	teaspoon ground nutmeg
3	cups uncooked Quaker Oats (quick or old-fashioned)

1. Preheat oven to 375° F.
2. In a large bowl, cream together margarine, brown sugar, and granulated sugar. Beat in the egg and vanilla. In a medium bowl, combine the flour, baking soda, salt, and spices. Add flour mixture into the wet ingredients and mix well. Stir in oats.
3. Drop by rounded tablespoonfuls onto an ungreased cookie sheet. Bake 8 to 9 minutes for a chewy cookie, 10 to 11 minutes for a crisp cookie. Cool 1 minute on cookie sheet, then remove to wire rack.

Makes 54 cookies.

*From the Quaker Oats Company. Used with permission.

**Nutrient Content
Per Serving (4 cookies)**   ★ **Star Rating: 2**   ❘ **Spoon Rating: 2**

Calories:	334 kcal	Vitamin A	20%	Egg
Protein:	5 g	Magnesium	20%	Oatmeal
Carbohydrate:	43 g			

Total Fat:	16 g
Saturated Fat:	9.6 g

Calcium:	75 mg
Iron:	1.9 mg

Dietary Fiber:	2.1 g

Fruit Crisp Delight *

¾ cup uncooked Quaker Oats (quick or old-fashioned)
¼ cup plus 3 tablespoons firmly packed brown sugar, divided
2 tablespoons margarine, melted
¼ teaspoon plus ½ teaspoon ground cinnamon, divided
6 cups peeled, thinly sliced apples, peaches, or pears (about 6 medium)
¼ cup water
2 tablespoons all-purpose flour

1. Preheat oven to 350° F.
2. In a large bowl, combine oats, 3 tablespoons firmly packed brown sugar, melted margarine, and ¼ teaspoon cinnamon; mix well.
3. In a large bowl, combine fruit and water. Add the ¼ cup brown sugar, flour, and ½ teaspoon cinnamon, tossing to coat. Spoon into 8-inch square glass baking dish and top with oat mixture. Bake 30 to 35 minutes or until fruit is tender.

Microwave Directions: Follow recipe as directed above, except spoon fruit mixture into microwavable baking dish; set aside oat mixture. Microwave on High for 6 minutes, stirring once. Top with reserved oat mixture. Microwave on High 3 to 6 minutes or until fruit is tender.
Makes 9 servings.

*From the Quaker Oats Company. Used with permission.

Nutrient Content Per Serving

★ Star Rating: 4   ⎮ Spoon Rating: 2

Calories:	194 kcal	Vitamin A	20%	Oatmeal	
Protein:	3 g	Vitamin C	22%	Apples	
Carbohydrate:	42 g	Vitamin E	20%		
		Fiber	20%		
Total Fat:	3 g				
Saturated Fat:	1 g				
Calcium:	25 mg				
Iron:	0.9 mg				
Dietary Fiber:	5.3 g				

Lemon Blueberry Muffins*

Topping
¼   cup uncooked Quaker oats (quick or old-fashioned)
2   tablespoons sugar

Muffins
     nonstick cooking spray
1½ cups uncooked Quaker Oats (quick or old-fashioned)
1   cup all-purpose flour
½   cup sugar
1   tablespoon baking powder
¼   teaspoon salt (optional)
1   cup skim milk
2   egg whites (or 1 egg, lightly beaten)
2   tablespoons safflower or canola oil
1   teaspoon vanilla extract
1   teaspoon grated lemon peel
1   cup fresh or frozen blueberries

1. Preheat oven to 400° F. Line 12 muffin cups with paper baking cups or spray bottoms only with nonstick cooking spray.
2. For topping, combine oats and sugar and set aside.
3. In a large bowl, combine oats, flour, sugar, baking powder, and salt. Mix in the milk, egg whites, oil, vanilla, and lemon peel just until dry ingredients are moistened. Gently stir in the blueberries.
4. Fill muffin cups ¾ full. Sprinkle with reserved topping, patting

*From the Quaker Oats Company. Used with permission.

gently. Bake 20 to 24 minutes or until light golden brown. Let muffins stand a few minutes; remove from pan. Serve warm. Makes 12 muffins.

Nutrient Content Per Serving		★ Star Rating: 3		Spoon Rating: 3
Calories:	320 kcal	Vitamin E	25%	Oatmeal
Protein:	8 g	Thiamin	22%	Milk
Carbohydrate:	57 g	Magnesium	25%	Eggs
Total Fat:	7 g			
Saturated Fat:	0.9 g			
Calcium:	70 mg			
Iron:	2.2 mg			
Dietary Fiber:	3.4 g			

Lemon Yogurt Cookies *

½ cup (1 stick) margarine, softened
1¼ cups granulated sugar
½ cup plain nonfat yogurt or lemon lowfat yogurt
2 egg whites (or 1 egg)
1 tablespoon grated lemon peel
½ teaspoon vanilla extract
2 cups uncooked Quaker Oats (quick or old-fashioned)
1½ cups all-purpose flour
1 teaspoon baking powder
½ teaspoon baking soda
   nonstick cooking spray
¼ cup powdered sugar

1. In a large bowl, cream together the margarine and sugar. Add the yogurt, egg whites, lemon peel, and vanilla and beat well. Add the oats, flour, baking powder, and baking soda and mix well. Cover and chill for 1 to 3 hours.

2. Preheat oven to 375° F. Lightly spray a cookie sheet with nonstick cooking spray. With lightly floured hands, shape dough into 1-inch balls; place on prepared cookie sheet. Flatten with the bottom of a glass dipped in water then in sugar. Bake 10 to 12 minutes or until the edges are lightly browned. Cool 2 minutes on the cookie sheet; then remove to a wire rack and allow to cool completely. Sprinkle the cookies with powdered sugar. Store tightly covered.

Makes 4 dozen cookies.

*From the Quaker Oats Company. Used with permission.

Nutrient Content
Per Serving (1 cookie)   ★ Star Rating: 0   Spoon Rating: 3

Calories:	69 kcal	Yogurt
Protein:	1.2 g	Eggs
Carbohydrate:	11 g	Oatmeal
Total Fat:	2 g	
Saturated Fat:	1.3 g	
Calcium:	8 mg	
Iron:	0.4 mg	
Dietary Fiber:	0.4 g	

Fruitful Morning Muesli *

2	cups uncooked Quaker Oats (quick or old-fashioned)
2	cups apple juice or apricot nectar
1½	cups any combination sliced fresh fruit, such as bananas, peaches, or strawberries
1	(8-ounce) carton vanilla lowfat yogurt
2	tablespoons chopped nuts (optional)

1. In a large bowl, combine all ingredients except nuts. Mix well.

2. Cover; refrigerate 8 hours or overnight. Serve cold; top with nuts, if desired. Refrigerate, covered, up to 4 days.

Makes 4 (1-cup) servings.

For extra flavor you can toast the nuts: Spread them evenly in a small, shallow baking pan and bake at 350° F for 5 to 8 minutes or until light golden brown, stirring occasionally. To toast in the microwave, spread the nuts on a microwave-safe plate. Microwave on High for 1 minute; stir. Continue microwaving, checking every 30 seconds, until nuts are crunchy.

Nutrient Content Per Serving		★ Star Rating: 4		🥄 Spoon Rating: 3
Calories:	282 kcal	Vitamin C	46%	Oatmeal
Protein:	10 g	Thiamin	20%	Yogurt
Carbohydrate:	50 g	Phosphorus	25%	Nuts
		Magnesium	45%	
Total Fat:	6 g			
Saturated Fat:	1 g			
Calcium:	141 mg			
Iron:	2.7 mg			
Dietary Fiber:	5.3 g			

*From the Quaker Oats Company. Used with permission.

Banana-Orange Oatmeal Muffins *

Nonstick cooking spray
1½ cups uncooked Quaker Oats (quick or old-fashioned)
1 cup all-purpose flour
⅓ cup firmly packed brown sugar
1 teaspoon baking powder
½ teaspoon baking soda
½ teaspoon ground cinnamon
¼ teaspoon salt (optional)
⅓ cup chopped dates or raisins
1 (8-ounce) carton plain nonfat yogurt or ¾ cup lowfat buttermilk
¾ cup mashed ripe banana (about 2 medium)
1 egg, lightly beaten
2 tablespoons safflower oil
1½ teaspoons grated orange peel

1. Preheat oven to 400° F. Line 12 medium muffin cups with paper liners or spray bottoms only with nonstick cooking spray.
2. In a large bowl, combine oats, flour, brown sugar, baking powder, baking soda, cinnamon, salt, and dates. Mix well.
3. In a medium bowl, combine the yogurt, banana, egg, oil, and orange peel. Pour mixture into the dry ingredients and mix just until moistened.
4. Fill prepared muffin cups ¾ full and bake 20 to 22 minutes or until golden brown. Let muffins stand a few minutes; remove from pan.
Makes 12 muffins.

*From the Quaker Oats Company. Used with permission.

**Nutrient Content
Per Serving**   ★ Star Rating: 3   ❘ Spoon Rating: 3

Calories:	305 kcal	Vitamin E	23%	Oatmeal
Protein:	7 g	Thiamin	20%	Yogurt
Carbohydrate:	54 g	Magnesium	25%	Eggs

Total Fat: 7 g
Saturated Fat: 3 g

Calcium: 67 mg
Iron: 2.4 mg

Dietary Fiber: 3.6 g

Wholesome
Apple-Raisin Muffins *

Nonstick cooking spray
1¾ cups uncooked Quaker Oats (quick or old-fashioned) divided
1 cup all-purpose flour
⅔ cup firmly packed brown sugar
1 teaspoon baking powder
½ teaspoon baking soda
½ teaspoon ground cinnamon
¼ teaspoon salt (optional)
½ cup raisins
¾ cup applesauce
⅓ cup skim milk
1 egg, lightly beaten
2 tablespoons safflower oil

1. Preheat oven to 400° F. Line 12 muffin cups with paper baking cups or spray bottoms only with nonstick cooking spray.
2. In a large bowl, combine 1½ cups oats, flour, brown sugar, baking powder, baking soda, cinnamon, salt, and raisins; mix well. Add the applesauce, skim milk, egg, and oil and mix just until dry ingredients are moistened.
3. Fill muffin cups ¾ full. Sprinkle with remaining ¼ cup oats, patting gently.
4. Bake 20 to 22 minutes or until golden brown. Let muffins stand a few minutes; remove from pan. Serve warm.
Makes 12 muffins.

*From the Quaker Oats Company. Used with permission.

Nutrient Content Per Serving   ★ **Star Rating: 3**   🥄 **Spoon Rating: 4**

Calories:	370 kcal	Vitamin E	23%	Oatmeal	
Protein:	7 g	Thiamin	22%	Apples	
Carbohydrate:	72 g	Magnesium	27%	Milk	
				Eggs	
Total Fat:	7 g				
Saturated Fat:	0.8 g				
Calcium:	62 mg				
Iron:	3 mg				
Dietary Fiber:	3.6 g				

Chewy Oatmeal Cookies*

¾   cup Butter Flavor Crisco shortening, plus enough to grease
    cookie sheet
1¼ cups firmly packed light brown sugar
1   egg
⅓   cup milk
1½ teaspoons vanilla extract
3   cups uncooked Quaker Oats (quick or old-fashioned)
1   cup all-purpose flour
½   teaspoon baking soda
½   teaspoon salt (optional)
¼   teaspoon cinnamon
1   cup raisins
1   cup coarsely chopped walnuts

1. Preheat oven to 375° F. Lightly grease a cookie sheet with Butter
   Flavor Crisco.
2. In a large bowl, combine ¾ cup Butter Flavor Crisco, brown
   sugar, egg, milk, and vanilla and beat with an electric mixer at
   medium speed until well blended.
3. Combine oats, flour, baking soda, salt, and cinnamon. Mix into
   batter at low speed just until blended. Stir in raisins and nuts.
4. Drop rounded tablespoonfuls of dough 2 inches apart onto
   prepared cookie sheet. Bake for 10 to 12 minutes or until lightly
   browned. Cool 2 minutes on cooling rack.

Makes 2½ dozen cookies.

*From the Quaker Oats Company. Used with permission.

Nutrient Content
Per Serving (1 cookie)   ★ Star Rating: 0   Spoon Rating: 4

Calories: 167 kcal   Egg
Protein: 3 g   Milk
Carbohydrate: 22 g   Oatmeal
                                   Nuts

Total Fat: 8 g
Saturated Fat: 1 g

Calcium: 25 mg
Iron: 1.1 mg

Dietary Fiber: 1.3 g

NOTES AND REFERENCES

C H A P T E R   1

1. Naeye, R.L., Blanc, W.A. & Paul, C. (1973). Effects of maternal nutrition on the human fetus. *Pediatrics* 52:494–503.
2. Barker, D.J., Bull, A.R., Osmond, C., et al. (1990). Fetal and placental size and risk of hypertension in adult life. *British Medical Journal* 301:259–262.
3. Wadsworth, M.E.J. & Kuh, D.J.L. (1997). Childhood influences on adult health: A review of recent work from the 1946 British national Birth Cohort study, MRC National Survey of Health and Development. *Paediatric and Perinatal Epidemiology* 11:2–20.
4. Neugebauer, R., Hoek, H.W. & Susser, E. (1999). Prenatal exposure to wartime famine and development of antisocial personality disorder in early adulthood. *Journal of the American Medical Association* 282:455–462.
5. Ravelli, G.P., Stein, Z.A. & Susser, M.W. (1976). Obesity in young men after famine exposure in utero and early infancy. *New England Journal of Medicine* 295:349–353.

Additional Studies of Interest

Barker, D.J.P. (1998). *Mothers, Babies and Health in Later Life* (2nd ed.). London: Churchill Livingstone.

C H A P T E R 2

1. Prasad, A.S. (1985). Clinical manifestations of zinc deficiency. *Annual Review of Nutrition* 5:341–363.

2. Keys A., Brozek, J., Henschel, A., Michelsen, O. & Taylor, H.L. (1950). *The Biology of Human Starvation.* Minneapolis, Mn.: University of Minnesota Press.

3. James, S.J., Pogribna, M., Pogribny, I.P., Melnyk, S., Hine, R.J., Gibson, J.B., Ping, Y., Tafoya, D.L., Swenson, D.H., Wilson, V.L. & Gaylor, D.W. (1999). Abnormal folate metabolism and mutation in the methylenetetrahydrofolate reductase gene may be maternal risk factors for Down syndrome. *American Journal of Clinical Nutrition* 70:495–501.

4. Rosenblatt, D.S. (1999). Folate and homocysteine metabolism and gene polymorphisms in the etiology of Down syndrome. *American Journal of Clinical Nutrition* 70:429–430.

5. Scholl, T.O., Hediger, M.L., Schall, J.I., Khoo, C.S. & Fischer, R.L. (1996). Dietary and serum folate: Their influence on the outcome of pregnancy. *American Journal of Clinical Nutrition* 63:520–5.

6. Centers for Disease Control (1992). Recommendations for use of folic acid to reduce number of spina bifida cases and other neural tube defects. *Morbidity and Mortality Weekly Report* 41RR–14.

7. Jacques P.F., Selhub, J., Bostom, A.G., Wilson, P.W.F. & Rosenberg, I.H. (1999). The effect of folic acid fortification on plasma folate and total homocysteine concentrations. *New England Journal of Medicine* 340:1449–1454.

8. Shaw, G.M., Lammer, E.J., Wasserman, C.R., O'Malley, C.D. & Tolarova, M.M. (1995). Risks of orofacial clefts in children born to women using multivitamins containing folic acid periconceptionally. *Lancet* 345:393–396.

9. Botto, L.D., Khoury, M.J., Mulinare, J. & Erickson, J.D. (1996). Periconceptional multivitamin use and the occurrence of conotruncal heart defects: Results from a population-based, case-control study. *Pediatrics* 98:911–917.

10. Botto, L.D., Mulinare, J. & Erickson, J.D. (2000). Occurrence of congenital heart defects in relation to maternal multivitamin use. *American Journal of Epidemiology* 151:878–884.

11. Czeizel, A.E. (1993). Prevention of congenital abnormalities by periconceptional multivitamin supplementation. *British Medical Journal* 306:1645–8.

12. Czeizel, A.E. (1996). Reduction of urinary tract and cardiovascular defects by periconceptional multivitamin supplementation. *American Journal of Medical Genetics* 62:179–183.

13. Li, D-K., Daling, J.R., Mueller, B.A., Hickok, D.E., Fantel, A.G. & Weiss, N.S. (1995). Periconceptional multivitamin use in relation to the risk of congenital urinary tract anomalies. *Epidemiology* 6:212–8.

14. Werler, M.M., Hayes, C., Louik, C., Shapiro, S. & Mitchell, A.A. (1999). Multivitamin supplementation and risk of birth defects. *American Journal of Epidemiology* 150:675–682.

15. Scholl, T.O., Hediger, M.L., Fischer, R.L. & Shearer, J.W. (1992). Anemia vs. iron deficiency: Increased risk of preterm delivery in a prospective study. *American Journal of Clinical Nutrition* 55:985–988.

16. Rushton, D.H. (1991). Ferritin and fertility (letter). *Lancet* 337:1554.

17. Enns, C.W., Goldman, J.D. & Cook, A. (1997). Trends in food and nutrient intakes by adults: NFCS 1977–78, CSFII 1989–91, and CSFII 1994–95. *Family Economics and Nutrition Review* 10:2–15.

18. Bolúmar, F., Olsen, J., Rebagliato, M., Saez-Lloret, I., Bisanti, L. & the European Study Group on Infertility and Subfecundity (2000). Body mass index and delayed conception: A European multicenter study on infertility and subfecundity. *American Journal of Epidemiology* 151:1072–9.

19. Cnattingius, S., Bergstrom, R., Lipworth, L. & Kramer, M.S. (1998). Prepregnancy weight and the risk of adverse pregnancy outcomes. *New England Journal of Medicine* 338:147–52.

20. Frisch, R.E. (1985). Fatness, menarche, and female fertility. *Perspectives in Biology and Medicine* 28:611–633.

21. Meyer, K.A., Kushi, L.H., Jacobs, D.R., Slavin, J., Sellers, T.A. & Folsom, A.R. (2000). Carbohydrates, dietary fiber, and incident type 2 diabetes in older women. *American Journal of Clinical Nutrition* 71:921–30.

22. Rimm, E.B., Willett, W.C., Hu, F.B., Sampson, L., Colditz, G.A., Manson, J.E., Hennekens, C. & Stampfer, M.J. (1998). Folate and vitamin B_6 from diet and supplements in relation to risk of coronary heart disease among women. *Journal of the American Medical Association* 279:359–364.

23. Morrison, H.I., Schaubel, D., Desmeules, M. & Wigle, D.T. (1996). Serum folate and risk of fatal coronary heart disease. *Journal of the American Medical Association* 275:1893–6.

24. Weir, D.G. & Molloy, A.M. (2000). Microvascular disease and dementia in the elderly: Are they related to hyperhomocysteinemia? *American Journal of Clinical Nutrition* 71:859–860.

Additional Studies of Interest

Belizàn, J.M., Villar, J., Gonzalez, L., Campodonico, L. & Bergel, E. (1991). Calcium supplementation to prevent hypertensive disorders of pregnancy. *New England Journal of Medicine* 325:1399–1405.

Bourgoin, B.P., Evans, D.R., Cornett, J.R., Lingard, S.M. & Quattrone, A.J. (1993). Lead content in 70 brands of dietary calcium supplements. *American Journal of Public Health* 83:1155–1160.

Brouwer, I.A., van Dusseldorp, M., Thomas, C.M.G., Duran, M., Hautvast, J.G.A.J., Eskes, T.K.A.B. & Steegers-Theunissen, R.P.M. (1999). Low-dose folic acid supplementation decreases plasma homocysteine concentrations: A randomized trial. *American Journal of Clinical Nutrition* 69:99–104.

Bucher, H.C., Guyatt, G.H., Cook, R.J., Hatala, R., Cook, D.J., Lang, J.D. & Hunt, D. (1996). Effect of calcium supplementation on pregnancy-induced hypertension and preeclampsia. *Journal of the American Medical Association* 275:1113–1117.

Dawson, E.B. (1986). Effect of ascorbic acid on male fertility. *Annals of the New York Academy of Sciences* 498:312–323.

Herrera, J.A., Arevalo-Herrera, M. & Herrera, S. (1998). Prevention of preeclampsia by linoleic acid and calcium supplementation: A randomized controlled trial. *Obstetrics and Gynecology* 91:585–90.

Levenson, D.I. & Bockman, R.S. (1994). A review of calcium preparations. *Nutrition Reviews* 52:221–232.

Picciano, M.F. (2000). Is homocysteine a biomarker for identifying women at risk of complications and adverse pregnancy outcomes? *American Journal of Clinical Nutrition* 71:857–8.

Riddell, L.J., Chisholm, A., Williams, S. & Mann, J.I. (2000). Dietary strategies for lowering homocysteine concentrations. *American Journal of Clinical Nutrition* 71:1448–1454.

Scholl, T.O., Hediger, M.L., Bendich, A., Schall, J.I., Smith, W.K. & Krueger, P.M. (1997). Use of multivitamin/mineral prenatal supplements: Influence on the outcome of pregnancy. *American Journal of Epidemiology* 146:134–141.

Seligman, P.A., Caskey, J.H., Frazier, J.L., Zucker, R.M., Podell, E.R. & Allen, R.H. (1983). Measurements of iron absorption from prenatal multivitamin-mineral supplements. *Obstetrics and Gynecology* 61:356–362.

Vollset, S.E., Refsum, H., Irgens, L.M., Emblem, B.M., Tverdal, A., Gjessing, H.K., Monsen, A.L.B. & Ueland, P.M. (2000). Plasma total homocysteine, pregnancy complications, and adverse pregnancy outcomes: the Hordaland Homocysteine Study. *American Journal of Clinical Nutrition* 71:962–8.

Whiting, S.J. (1994). Safety of some calcium supplements questioned. *Nutrition Reviews* 52:95–105.

C H A P T E R   3

1. Waisbren, S.E., Hanley, W. & Levy, H.L. (2000). Outcome at age 4 years in offspring of women with maternal phenylketonuria: The maternal PKU collaborative study. *Journal of the American Medical Association* 283:756–762.

2. Ebrahim, S.H., Floyd, R.L., Merritt, R.K., Decoufle, P. & Holtzman, D. (2000). Trends in pregnancy-related smoking rates in the United States, 1987–1996. *Journal of the American Medical Association* 283:361–6.

3. Armstrong, B.G., McDonald, A.D. & Sloan, M. (1992). Cigarette, alcohol, and coffee consumption and spontaneous abortion. *American Journal of Public Health* 82:85–87.

4. Källén, K. (2000). Multiple malformations and maternal smoking. *Paediatric and Perinatal Epidemiology* 14:227–233.

5. D'Souza, S.W., Black, P. & Richards, B. (1981). Smoking in pregnancy: Associations with skinfold thickness, maternal weight gain, and fetal size at birth. *British Medical Journal* 282:998–1000.

6. Peacock, J.L., Bland, J.M. & Anderson, H.R. (1995). Preterm delivery: Effects of socioeconomic factors, psychological stress, smoking, alcohol, and caffeine. *British Medical Journal* 311:531–5.

7. Shaw, N.R. & Bracken, M.B. (2000). A systematic review and meta-analysis of prospective studies on the association between maternal cigarette smoking and preterm delivery. *American Journal of Obstetrics and Gynecology* 182:465–472.

8. Olds, D. (1994). Intellectual impairment in children of women who smoke cigarettes during pregnancy. *Pediatrics* 93:221–7.

9. Tuthill, D.P., Stewart, J.H., Coles, E.C., Andrews, J. & Cartlidge, P.H.T. (1999). Maternal cigarette smoking and pregnancy outcome. *Paediatric and Perinatal Epidemiology* 13:245–253.

10. Savitz, D. (1991). Prenatal exposure to parent's smoking and child-hood cancer. *American Journal of Epidemiology* 133:123–132.

11. Ogburn, P.L., Hurt, R.D., Croghan, I.T., Schroeder, D.R., Ramin, K.D., Offord, K.P. & Moyer, T.P. (1999). Nicotine patch use in pregnant smokers: Nicotine and cotinine levels and fetal effects. *American Journal of Obstetrics and Gynecology* 181:736–743.

12. Dejin-Karlsson, E., Hanson, B.S., Östergren, P-O., Sjöberg, N-O. & Marsal, K. (1998). Does passive smoking in early pregnancy increase the risk of small-for-gestational-age infants? *American Journal of Public Health* 88:1523–7.

13. Hughes, E.G. & Brennan, B.G. (1996). Does cigarette smoking impair natural or assisted fecundity? *Fertility and Sterility* 66:679–689.

14. Lemoine, P., Harrousseau, M., Borteyru, J.P. et al. (1968) Les enfants de parents alcooliques: anomalies observées. *Ouest Med* 21:476–482.

15. Jones, K.L. & Smith, A.W. (1973). Recognition of the fetal alcohol syndrome in early infancy. *Lancet* 2:999–1001.

16. Larroque, B., Kaminski, M., Dehaene, P., Subtil, D., Delfosse, M-J. & Querleu, D. (1995). Moderate prenatal alcohol exposure and psychomotor development at preschool age. *American Journal of Public Health* 85:1654–61.

17. Windham, G.C., Fenster, L., Hopkins, B. & Swan, S.H. (1995). The association of moderate maternal and paternal alcohol consumption with birthweight and gestational age. *Epidemiology* 6:591–7.

18. Centers for Disease Control (1997). Alcohol consumption among pregnant and childbearing-aged women—United States, 1991 and 1995. *Morbidity and Mortality Weekly Report* 46:346–350.

19. Ebrahim, S.H., Luman, E.T., Floyd, R.L., Murphy, C.C., Bennett, E.M. & Boyle, C.A. (1998). Alcohol consumption by pregnant women in the United States during 1988–1995. *Obstetrics and Gynecology* 92:187–92.

20. Ebrahim, S.H., Diekman, S.T., Floyd, R.L. & Decoufle, P. (1999). Comparison of binge drinking among pregnant and nonpregnant women, United States, 1991–1995. *American Journal of Obstetrics and Gynecology* 180:1–7.

21. Fenster, L., et al. (1991). Caffeine consumption during pregnancy and fetal growth. *American Journal of Public Health* 81:458–461.

22. Infante-Rivard, C. et al. (1993). Fetal loss associated with caffeine intake before and after pregnancy. *Journal of the American Medical Association* 270:2940–3.

23. Wilcox A., et al. (1988). Caffeinated beverages and decreased fertility. *Lancet 2* (8626–8627):1453–6.
24. Williams, M.A., Mittendorf, R., Stubblefield, P.G., Lieberman, E., Schoenbaum, S.C. & Monson, R.R. (1992). Cigarettes, coffee, and preterm premature rupture of the membranes. *American Journal of Epidemiology* 135:895–903.
25. Dlugosz, L., Belanger, K., Hellenbrand, K., Holford, T.R., Leaderer, B., Bracken, M.B. (1996). Maternal caffeine consumption and spontaneous abortion: A prospective cohort study. *Epidemiology* 7:250–5.
26. Cook, A.J.C., Gilbert, R.E., Buffolano, W., et al. (2000). Sources of toxoplasma infection in pregnant women: European multicentre case-control study. *British Medical Journal* 321:142–7.
27. Dubey, J.P. (2000). Sources of *Toxoplasma gondii* infection in pregnancy. *British Medical Journal* 321:127–8.

Additional Studies of Interest

Luke, B., & Keith, L.G. (1990). The challenge of maternal phenylketonuria screening and treatment. *Journal of Reproductive Medicine* 35:667–673.
Mills, J.L., Graubard, B.I., Harley, E.E., Rhoads, G.G. & Berends, H.W. (1984). Maternal alcohol consumption and birth weight: How much drinking in pregnancy is safe? *Journal of the American Medical Association* 252:1875–9.

C H A P T E R   4

1. American College of Obstetricians and Gynecologists (2000). *Planning for Pregnancy, Birth, and Beyond,* 3rd ed.
2. Hadlock, F.P., Deter, R.L., Harrist, R.B., Roecker, E. & Park, S.K. (1983). A date-independent predictor of intrauterine growth retardation: Femur length/abdominal circumference ratio. *American Journal of Radiology* 141:979–984.
3. Westgren, M., Beall, M., Divon, M. & Platt, L. (1986). Fetal femur length/abdominal circumference ratio in preterm labor patients with and without successful tocolytic therapy. *Journal of Ultrasound in Medicine* 5:243–5.
4. Hediger, M.L., Scholl, T.O., Schall, J.I., Miller, L.W. & Fischer, R.L. (1995). Fetal growth and the etiology of preterm delivery. *Obstetrics and Gynecology* 85:175–182.
5. Campbell, S. & Thoms, A. (1977). Ultrasound measurement of the fetal head to abdomen circumference in the assessment of growth retardation. *British Journal of Obstetrics and Gynaecology* 84:165–174.

6. Ott, W.J. (1993). Intrauterine growth retardation and preterm delivery. *American Journal of Obstetrics and Gynecology* 168:1710–1717.

7. Weiner, C.P., Sabbagha, R.E., Vaisrub, N. & Depp, R. (1985). A hypothetical model suggesting suboptimal intrauterine growth in infants delivered preterm. *Obstetrics and Gynecology* 65:323–326.

8. MacGregor, S.N., Sabbagha, R.E., Tamura, R.K., Pielet, B.W. & Feigenbaum, S.L. (1988). Differing fetal growth patterns in pregnancies complicated by preterm labor. *Obstetrics and Gynecology* 72:834–837.

9. Phillips, D.I.W., Cooper, C., Fall, C., Prentice, L., Osmond, C., Barker, D.J.P. & Rees Smith, B. (1993). Fetal growth and autoimmune thyroid disease. *Quarterly Journal of Medicine* 86:247–253.

10. Godfrey, K.M., Barker, D.J.P. & Osmond, C. (1994). Disproportionate fetal growth and raised IgE concentration in adult life. *Clinical and Experimental Allergy* 24:641–648.

11. Fergusson, D.M., Crane, J., Beasley, R. & Horwood, L.J. (1997). Perinatal factors and atopic disease in childhood. *Clinical and Experimental Allergy* 27:1394–1401.

CHAPTER 5

1. Huxley, R.R. (2000). Nausea and vomiting in early pregnancy: Its role in placental development. *Obstetrics and Gynecology* 95:779–82.

2. Kdllin, B. (1987). Hyperemesis during pregnancy and delivery outcome: A registry study. *European Journal of Obstetrics and Gynaecology and Reproductive Biology* 26:291–302.

3. Deuchar, N. (1995). Nausea and vomiting in pregnancy: A review of the problem with particular regard to psychological and social aspects. *British Journal of Obstetrics and Gynaecology* 102:6–8.

4. Godsey, R. (1991). Hyperemesis gravidarum: A comparison of single and multiple admissions. *Journal of Reproductive Medicine* 36:287–290.

5. Gross, S. (1989). Maternal weight loss associated with hyperemesis gravidarum: A predictor of fetal outcome. *American Journal of Obstetrics and Gynecology* 160:906–9.

6. van Stuijvenberg, M.E., Schabort, I., Labadarios, D. & Nel, J.T. (1995). The nutritional status and treatment of patients with hyperemesis gravidarum. *American Journal of Obstetrics and Gynecology* 172:1585–91.

Additional Studies of Interest

Behrman, C. (1990). Nausea and vomiting during teenage pregnancy: Effects on birth weight. *Journal of Adolescent Health Care* 11:418–422.

Klebanoff, M.A., Koslowe, P.A., Kaslow, R. & Rhoads, G.G. (1985). Epidemiology of vomiting in early pregnancy. *Obstetrics and Gynecology* 66:612–616.

Tsang, I.S., Katz, V.L. & Wells, S.D. (1996). Maternal and fetal outcomes in hyperemesis gravidarum. *International Journal of Gynaecology and Obstetrics* 55:231–235.

Weigel, R. & Weigel, M. (1989). Nausea and vomiting of early pregnancy and pregnancy outcome: A meta-analytical review. *British Journal of Obstetrics and Gynaecology* 96:1312–1318.

C H A P T E R   6

1. Hadders-Algra, M. & Touwen, B.C.L. (1990). Body measurements, neurological and behavioral development in six-year-old children born preterm and/or small for gestational age. *Early Human Development* 22:1–13.

2. Parkinson, C.E., Scrivener, R., Graves, L., Bunton, J. & Harvey, D. (1986). Behavioral differences of school age children who were small for dates babies. *Developmental Medicine and Child Neurology* 28:498–505.

3. Rubin, R.A., Rosenblatt, C. & Balow, B. (1973). Physiology and educational sequelae of prematurity. *Pediatrics* 52:352–363.

4. Francois, I., de Zegher, F., Spiessens, C., D'Hooghe, T. & Vander-Schueren, D. (1997). Low birth weight and subsequent male subfertility. *Pediatric Research* 42:899–901.

5. Plante, L.A. (1998). Small size at birth and later diabetic pregnancy. *Obstetrics and Gynecology* 92:781–4.

6. Paz, I., Gale, R., Laor, A., Danon, Y.L., Stevenson, D.K. & Seidman, D.S. (1995). The cognitive outcome of full-term small for gestational age infants at late adolescence. *Obstetrics and Gynecology* 85:452–6.

7. Sørensen, H.T., Sabroe, S., Olsen, J., Rothman, K.J., Gillman, M.W. & Fischer, P., et al (1997). Birth weight and cognitive function in young adult life. *British Medical Journal* 316:401–3.

8. Strauss, R.S. (2000). Adult functional outcome of those born small for gestational age: Twenty-six year follow-up of the 1970 British Birth Cohort. *Journal of the American Medical Association* 283:625–632.

9. Paz, I., Seidman, D.S., Danon, Y.L., Laor, A., Stevenson, D.K. & Gale, R. (1993). Are children born small for gestational age at increased risk for short stature? *American Journal of Diseases of Children* 147:337–9.

10. Scholl, T.O., Hediger, M.L., Bendich, A., Schall, J.I., Smith, W.K. & Krueger, P.M. (1997). Use of multivitamin/mineral prenatal supplements: Influence on the outcome of pregnancy. *American Journal of Epidemiology* 146:134–141.

11. O'Connell, M. (1991). Maternity leave arrangements: 1961–85. In: Work and family patterns of American women, June, 1990. Washington, D.C.: U.S. Govt. Printing Office.

12. Mozurkewich, E.L., Luke, B., Avni, M. & Wolf, F.M. (2000). Working conditions and adverse pregnancy outcome: A meta-analysis. *Obstetrics and Gynecology* 95:623–35.

13. Luke, B., Avni, M., Min, L. & Misiunas, R. (1999). Work and pregnancy: The role of fatigue and the "second shift" on antenatal morbidity. *American Journal of Obstetrics and Gynecology* 181:1172–9.

14. Luke, B., Mamelle, N., Keith, L., Munoz, F., Minogue, J., Papiernik, E. & Johnson, T.R.B. (1995). The association between occupational factors and preterm birth: A United States nurses' study. *American Journal of Obstetrics and Gynecology* 173:849–62.

15. Luke, B. & Eberlein, T. (1999). *When You're Expecting Twins, Triplets, or Quads.* HarperCollins: New York.

Additional Studies of Interest

Barker, D.J.P., Martyn, C.N., Osmond, C., Wield, G.A. (1995). Abnormal liver growth in utero and death from coronary heart disease. *British Medical Journal* 310:703–4.

Barker, D.J.P., Osmond, C. & Golding, J. (1990). Height and mortality in the countries of England and Wales. *Annals of Human Biology* 17:1–6.

Ekbom, A., Hsieh, C.C., Lipworth, L., et al. (1996). Perinatal characteristics in relation to incidence of and mortality from prostate cancer. *British Medicine Journal* 313:337–341.

Michels, K.B., Trichopoulos, D., Robins, J.M., et al. (1996). Birthweight as a risk factor for breast cancer. *Lancet* 348:1542–6.

CHAPTER 7

1. Hediger, M.L., Overpeck, M.D., Kuczmarski, R.J., McGlynn, A., Maurer, K.R. & Davis, W.W. (1998). Muscularity and fatness of infants and young children born small- or large-for-gestational age. *Pediatrics* 102: e60.

2. Yau, K.I. & Chang, M.H. (1993). Growth and body composition of preterm, small-for-gestational-age infants at a postmenstrual age of 37–40 weeks. *Early Human Development* 33:117–131.

3. Hay, W.W. Jr., Catz, C.S., Grave, G.D. & Yaffe, S.J. (1997). Fetal growth: Its regulation and disorders. *Pediatrics* 99:585–591.
4. de Groot, L., de Groot, C.J., Hopkins, B. (1997). An instrument to measure independent walking: Are there differences between preterm and fullterm infants? *Journal of Child Neurology* 12:37–41.
5. Hofman, P.O.L., Cutfield, W.S. & Robinson, E.M. (1997). Insulin resistance in short children with intrauterine growth retardation. *Journal of Clinical Endocrinology and Metabolism* 82:402–6.
6. Gambacciani, M., Spinetti, A., Gallo, R., Cappagli, B., Teti, G.C. & Facchini, V. (1995). Ultrasonographic bone characteristics during normal pregnancy: Longitudinal and cross-sectional evaluation. *American Journal of Obstetrics and Gynecology* 173:890–3.
7. Okah, F.A., Tsang, R.C., Sierra, R., Brady, K.K. & Specker, B.L. (1996). Bone turnover and mineral metabolism in the last trimester of pregnancy: Effect of multiple gestation. *Obstetrics and Gynecology* 88:168–73.
8. Koo, W.W.K., Walters, J.C., Esterlitz, J., Levine, R.J., Bush, A.J. & Sibai, B. (1999). Maternal calcium supplementation and fetal bone mineralization. *Obstetrics and Gynecology* 94:577–82.
9. Rizzo, T., Metzger, B.E., Burns, W.J. & Burns, K. (1991). Correlations between antepartum maternal metabolism and intelligence of offspring. *New England Journal of Medicine* 325:911–6.
10. Rizzo, T.A., Dooley, S.L., Metzger, B.E., Cho, N.H., Ogata, E.S. & Silverman, B.L. (1995). Prenatal and perinatal influences on long-term psychomotor development in offspring of diabetic mothers. *American Journal of Obstetrics and Gynecology* 173:1753–8.
11. Rizzo, T., Freinkel, N., Metzger, B.E., Hatcher, R., Burns, W.J. & Barglow, P. (1990). Correlations between antepartum maternal metabolism and newborn behavior. *American Journal of Obstetrics and Gynecology* 163:1458–64.
12. Petersen, M.B., Pedersen, S.A., Greisen, G., Pedersen, J.F. & Molsted-Pedersen, L. (1988). Early growth delay in diabetic pregnancy: Relation to psychomotor development at age 4. *British Medical Journal* 296:598–600.
13. Churchill, J.A., Berendes, H.W. & Nemore, J. (1969). Neuropsychological deficits in children of diabetic mothers: A report from the Collaborative Study of Cerebral Palsy. *American Journal of Obstetrics and Gynecology* 105:257–268.
14. Stehbens, J.A., Baker, G.L. & Kitchell, M. (1977). Outcome at ages 1,

3, and 5 years of children born to diabetic women. *American Journal of Obstetrics and Gynecology* 127:408–413.

15. Marcoux, S., Brisson, J. & Fabia, J. (1991). Calcium intake from dairy products and supplements and the risks of preeclampsia and gestational hypertension. *American Journal of Epidemiology* 133:1266–72.

16. Belizàn, J.M., Villar, J., Gonzalez, L., Campodonico, L. & Bergel, E. (1991). Calcium supplementation to prevent hypertensive disorders of pregnancy. *New England Journal of Medicine* 325:1399–1405.

17. Herrera, J.A., Arevalo-Herrera, M. & Herrera, S. (1998). Prevention of preeclampsia by linoleic acid and calcium supplementation: A randomized controlled trial. *Obstetrics and Gynecology* 91:585–90.

18. Bucher, H.C., Guyatt, G.H., Cook, R.J., Hatala, R., Cook, D.J., Lang, J.D. & Hunt, D. (1996). Effect of calcium supplementation on pregnancy-induced hypertension and preeclampsia. *Journal of the American Medical Association* 275:1113–7.

19. Wacker, J., Frühauf, J., Schulz, M., Chiwora, F.M., Volz, J. & Becker, K. (2000). Riboflavin deficiency and preeclampsia. *Obstetrics and Gynecology* 96:38–44.

20. Oomen, C.M., Feskens, E.J.M., Räsänen, L., Fidanza, F., Nissinen, A.M., Menotti, A., Kok, F.J. & Kromhout, D. (2000). Fish consumption and coronary heart disease mortality in Finland, Italy, and the Netherlands. *American Journal of Epidemiology* 151:999–1006.

21. Shapiro, J.A., Koepsell, T.D., Voigt, L.F., Dugowson, C.E., Kestin, M. & Nelson, J.L. (1996). Diet and rhematoid arthritis in women: A possible protective effect of fish consumption. *Epidemiology* 7:256–263.

Additional Studies of Interest

Barker, D.J.P. (1998). *Mothers, Babies and Health in Later Life* (2nd ed). London: Churchill Livingstone.

Cresswell, J.L., Egger, P., Fall, C.H.D., Osmond, C., Fraser, R.B. & Barker, D.J.P. (1997). Is the age of menopause determined in-utero? *Early Human Development* 49:143–148.

CHAPTER 8

1. O'Shea, T.M., Klinepeter, K.L., Meis, P.J. & Dillard, R.G. (1998). Intrauterine infection and the risk of cerebral palsy in very low-birthweight infants. *Paediatric and Perinatal Epidemiology* 12:72–83.

2. Barker, D.J.P., Osmond, C., Rodin, I., Fall, C.H.D. & Winter, P.D. (1995). Low weight gain in infancy and suicide in adult life. *British Medical Journal* 311:1203.

3. Shaheen, S.O. & Barker. D.J.P. (1994). Early lung growth and chronic airflow obstruction. *Thorax* 49:533–6.

4. Hoffman, H.J. & Hillman, L.S. (1992). Epidemiology of the sudden infant death syndrome: Maternal, neonatal, and postneonatal risk factors. *Clinical Perinatology* 19:717–737.

5. Malloy, M.H. & Hoffman, H.J. (1995) Prematurity, sudden infant death syndrome, and age of death. *Pediatrics* 96:464–471.

6. Schoendorf, K.C. & Kiely, J.L. (1992). Relationship of sudden infant death syndrome to maternal smoking during and after pregnancy. *Pediatrics* 90:905–8.

7. Lucas, A., Morley, R., Cole, T.J., Lister, G. & Leeson-Payne, C. (1992). Breast milk and subsequent intelligence quotient in children born pre-term. *Lancet* 339:261–4.

8. Horwood, L.J. & Fergusson, D.M. (1998). Breastfeeding and later cognitive and academic outcomes. *Pediatrics* 101:1–7.

9. Lucas, A., Morley, R. & Cole, T.J. (1998). Randomized trial of early diet in preterm babies and later intelligence. *British Medical Journal* 317:1481–7.

10. Newacheck, P.W. & Halfon, N. (2000). Prevalence, impact, and trends in childhood disability due to asthma. *Archives of Pediatric and Adolescent Medicine* 154:287–293.

11. Oddy, W.H., Holt, P.G., Sly, P.D. et al. (1999). Association between breast feeding and asthma in 6 year old children: Findings of a prospective birth cohort study. *British Medical Journal* 319:815–9.

12. Aniansson, G., Alm, B., Andersson, B. et al. (1994). A prospective cohort study on breastfeeding and otitis media in Swedish infants. *Pediatric Infectious Disease Journal* 13:183–188.

13. Teele, D.W., Klein, J.O. & Rosner, B. (1989). Epidemiology of otitis media during the first seven years of life in children in greater Boston: A prospective, cohort study. *Journal of Infectious Disease* 169:83–94.

14. Howie, P.W., Forsyth, J.S., Ogston, S.A., Clark, A. & du V Florey, C. (1990). Protective effect of breastfeeding against infection. *British Medical Journal* 300:11–16.

15. Raisler, J., Alexander, C. & O'Campo, P. (1999). Breast-feeding and infant illness: A dose-response relationship? *American Journal of Public Health* 89:25–30.

16. Dewey, K.G., Heinig, M.J. & Nommsen, L.A. (1993). Maternal weight-loss patterns during prolonged lactation. *American Journal of Clinical Nutrition* 58:162–6.

17. Kramer, F.M., Stunkard, A.J., Marshall, K.A., McKinney, S. & Lieb-schutz, J. (1993). Breast-feeding reduces maternal lower-body fat. *Journal of the American Dietetic Association* 93:429–433.

18. Hediger, M.L., Overpeck, M.D., Ruan, W.J. & Troendle, J.F. (2000). Early infant feeding and growth status of US-born infants and children aged 4–71 mo: Analyses from the third National Health and Nutrition Examination Survey, 1988–1994. *American Journal of Clinical Nutrition* 72:159–167.

19. Hibbeln, J.R. & Salem, N. (1995). Dietary polyunsaturated fatty acids and depression: When cholesterol does not satisfy. *American Journal of Clinical Nutrition* 62:1–9.

20. Wilson, A.C., Forsyth, J.S., Greene, S.A., Irvine, L. & Hau, C. (1998). Relation of infant diet to childhood health: Seven year follow up of cohort of children in Dundee infant feeding study. *British Medical Journal* 316:21–25.

21. Satter, E. (1987). *How to Get Your Child to Eat—But Not Too Much.* Palo Alto, Calif.: Bull Publishing.

22. Albertsson-Wikland, K., Wennergren, G., Wennergren, M., Vilbergs-son, G. & Rosberg, S. (1993). Longitudinal follow-up of growth in children born small for gestational age. *Acta Paediatrica Scandinavia* 82:438–443.

23. Tenovuo, A., Kero, P., Piekkala, P., Korvenrata, H., Sillanpaa, M. & Erkkola, R. (1987). Growth of 519 small-for-gestational-age infants during the first two years of life. *Acta Paediatrica Scandinavia* 76:636–646.

24. Karlberg, J. & Albertsson-Wikland, K. (1995). Growth in full-term small-for-gestational-age infants: From birth to final height. *Pediatric Research* 38:1–7.

25. Berlin, U., Brooks-Gunn, J., McCarton, C. & McCormick, M.C. (1998). The effectiveness of early intervention: Examining risk factors and pathways to enhanced development. *Preventive Medicine* 27:238–245.

26. Weikart, D.P. (1998). Changing early childhood development through educational intervention. *Preventive Medicine* 27:233–237.

27. Strauss, R.S. (2000). Adult functional outcome of those born small for gestational age: Twenty-six-year follow-up of the 1970 British Birth Cohort. *Journal of the American Medical Association* 283:625–632.

28. Rosenblatt, K.A. & Thomas, D.B. (1993). WHO collaborative study of neoplasia and steroid contraceptives. *International Journal of Epidemiology* 22:192–197.

29. United Kingdom National Case-Control Study Group (1993). Breast

feeding and risk of breast cancer in young women. *British Medical Journal* 307:17–20.

30. Newcomb, P.A., Storer, B.E., Longnecker, M.P. et al. (1994). Lactation and reduced risk of premenopausal breast cancer. *New England Journal of Medicine* 330:81–87.

31. Kalkwarf, H.J. & Specker, B.L. (1995). Bone mineral loss during lactation and recovery after weaning. *Obstetrics and Gynecology* 86:26–32.

32. Specker, B.L., Tsang, R.C. & Ho, M.L. (1991). Changes in calcium homeostasis over the first year postpartum: Effect of lactation and weaning. *Obstetrics and Gynecology* 78:56–61.

33. Sowers, M.F., Corton, G., Shapiro, B. et al. (1993). Changes in bone density with lactation. *Journal of the American Medical Association* 269:3130–5.

34. Sowers, M.F., Randolph, J., Shapiro, B. & Jannausch, M. (1995). A prospective study of bone density and pregnancy after an extended period of lactation with bone loss. *Obstetrics and Gynecology* 85:285–9.

35. Laskey, M.A., Prentice, A., Hanratty, L.A., Jarjou, L.M.A., Dibba, B., Beavan, S.R. & Cole, T.J. (1998). Bone changes after 3 months of lactation: Influence of calcium intake, breast milk output, and vitamin D-receptor genotype. *American Journal of Clinical Nutrition* 67:685–692.

36. Polatti, F., Capuzzo, E., Viazzo, F. Colleoni, R. & Klersy, C. (1999). Bone mineral changes during and after lactation. *Obstetrics and Gynecology* 94:52–6.

37. Aihie, S.A., Cooper, C. & Barker, D.J.P. (1997). Is life span determined in utero? *Archives of Diseases of Children* 77:F161–F162.

Additional Studies of Interest

Karlberg, J.P.E., Albertsson-Wikland, K., Kwan, E.Y.W., Lam, B.C.C. & Low, L.C.K. (1997). The timing of early postnatal catch-up growth in normal, full-term infants born short for gestational age. *Hormonal Research* 48:17–24.

C H A P T E R   9

1. Anderson, R.N. (1999). United States life tables, 1997. *National Vital Statistics Reports,* 28.

2. Ounsted, M., Moar, V. & Scott, A. (1982). Growth in the first four years: II. Diversity within groups of small-for-dates and large-for-dates babies. *Early Human Development* 7:29–39.

3. Van Cauter, E., Leproult, R. & Plat, L. (2000). Age-related changes in slow wave sleep and REM sleep and relationship with growth hormone and cortisol levels in healthy men. *Journal of the American Medical Association* 284:861–8.

4. Blackman, M.R. (2000). Age-related alterations in sleep quality and neuroendocrine function. *Journal of the American Medical Association* 284:879–881.

5. Eberlein, T. (1996). *Sleep: How to Teach Your Child to Sleep Like a Baby.* Pocket Books: New York.

6. U.S. Department of Agriculture, Agricultural Research Service (1999). Food and nutrient intakes by children 1994–96, 1998. Online at ARS Food Surveys Research Group and available on the Products page at www.barc.usda.gov/bharc/foodsurvey.

7. Committee on Nutrition, American Academy of Pediatrics (1998). Cholesterol in childhood. Policy Statement.

8. Ellison, R.C., Singer, M.R., Moore, L.L., et al. (1995). Current caffeine intake of young children: Amount and sources. *Journal of the American Medical Association* 95:802–4.

9. Litovitz, T.L., Holm, K.C., Bailey, K.M. & Schmitz, B.F. (1992). 1991 Annual report of the American Association of Poison Control Centers National Data Collection System. *American Journal of Emergency Medicine* 10:452–505.

10. (1994). Prevalence of overweight among adolescents—United States, 1988–91. *Morbidity and Mortality Weekly Report* 43:818–21.

11. (1997). Update: Prevalence of overweight among children, adolescents, and adults—United States, 1988–1994. *Morbidity and Mortality Weekly Report* 46:199–202.

12. (1998). Prevalence of overweight among third- and sixth-grade children—New York City, 1996. *Morbidity and Mortality Weekly Report* 47:980–984.

13. Troiano, R.P. & Flegal, K.M. (1998). Overweight children and adolescents: Description, epidemiology, and demographics. *Pediatrics* 101:497–504.

14. Mokdad, A.H., Serdula, M.K., Dietz, W.H., Bowman, B.A., Marks, J.S. & Koplan, J.P. (1999). The spread of the obesity epidemic in the United States, 1991–1998. *Journal of the American Medical Association* 282:1519–1522.

15. Must, A., Spadano, J., Coakley, E.H., Field, A.E., Colditz, G. & Dietz,

W.H. (1999). The disease burden associated with overweight and obesity. *Journal of the American Medical Association* 282:1523–1529.

16. Huang, Z., Willett, W.C., Manson, J.A.E., et al. (1998). Body weight, weight change, and risk for hypertension in women. *Annals of Internal Medicine* 128:81–88.

17. Stevens, J., Cai, J., Pamuk, E.R., et al. (1998). The effect of age on the association between body-mass index and mortality. *New England Journal of Medicine* 338:1–7.

18. Ravelli, G-P., Stein, Z.A. & Susser, M.W. (1976). Obesity in young men after famine exposure in utero and early infancy. *New England Journal of Medicine* 295:349–353.

19. Ravelli, A.C.J., van der Meulen, J.H.P., Osmond, C., Barker, D.J.P. & Bleker, O.P. (1999). Obesity at the age of 50 years in men and women exposed to famine prenatally. *American Journal of Clinical Nutrition* 70:811–816.

20. Leon, D.A., Koupilova, I., Lithell, H.O. et al. (1996). Failure to realize growth potential in utero and adult obesity in relation to blood pressure in 50-year-old Swedish men. *British Medical Journal* 312:401–6.

21. Barker, D.J.P. (1998) *Mothers, Babies and Health in Later Life* (2nd ed.). London: Churchill Livingstone.

22. Valdez, R., Athens, M.A., Thompson, G.H., Bradshaw, B.S. & Stern, M.P. (1994). Birthweight and adult health outcomes in a biethnic population in the USA. *Diabetologia* 37:624–631.

23. Barker, D.J., Meade, T.W., Fall, C.H., et al. (1992). Relation of fetal and infant growth to plasma fibrinogen and factor VII concentrations in adult life. *British Medical Journal* 304:148–152.

24. Martyn, C.N., Meade, T.W., Stirling, Y., et al. (1995). Plasma concentrations of fibrinogen and factor VII in adult life and their relation to intra-uterine growth. *British Journal of Haematology* 89:142–6.

25. Cook, D.G., Whincup, P.H., Miller, G., Carey, I., Adshead, F.J., Papacosta, O., Walker, M. & Howarth, D. (1999). Fibrinogen and factor VII levels are related to adiposity but not fetal growth or social class in children aged 10–11 years. *American Journal of Epidemiology* 150:727–736.

26. Guo, S.S., Roche, A.F., Chumlea, W.C., Gardner, J.D. & Siervogel, R.M. (1994). The predictive value of childhood body mass index values for overweight at age 35 years. *American Journal of Clinical Nutrition* 59:810–9.

27. Abraham, S. & Nordseick, M. (1960). Relationship of excess weight in children and adults. *Public Health Report* 75:263–273.

28. Kolata, G. (1986). Obese children: A growing problem. *Science* 232:20–1.

29. Whitaker, R.C., Wright J.A., Pepe, M.S., Seidel, K.D. & Dietz, W.H. (1997). Predicting obesity in young adulthood from childhood and parental obesity. *New England Journal of Medicine* 337:869–873.

30. Committee on Sports Medicine and Fitness. (1992). Fitness, activity, and sports participation in the preschool child. *Pediatrics* 90:1002–4.

31. Simon, J.A., Morrison, J.A., Similo, S.L., McMahon, R.P. & Schreiber, G.B. (1995). Correlates of high-density lipoprotein cholesterol in black girls and white girls: the NHLBI growth and health study. *American Journal of Public Health* 85:1698–1702.

32. Koval, J.A., DeFronzo, R.A., O'Doherty, R.M., Printz, R., Ardehali, H., Granner, D.K. & Mandarino, L.J. (1998). Regulation of hexokinase II activity and expression in human muscle by moderate exercise. *American Journal of Physiology* 274:E304–E308.

33. Nieman, D.C. (1997). Immune response to heavy exertion. *Journal of Applied Physiology* 82:1385–94.

34. Hahn, R.A., Teutsch, S.M., Rothenberg, R.B. & Marks, J.S. (1986). Excess deaths from nine chronic diseases in the United States. *Journal of the American Medical Association* 264:2654–9.

35. McGinnis, J.M. & Foege, W.H. (1993). Actual causes of death in the United States. *Journal of the American Medical Association* 270:2207–12.

36. U.S. Department of Health and Human Services. (1986). 1985 President's council on physical fitness and sports youth fitness survey. Washington, D.C.: U.S. Government Printing Office.

37. Persson, I., Ahlsson, F., Ewald, U., et al. (1999). Influence of perinatal factors on the onset of puberty in boys and girls: Implications for interpretation of link with risk of long term diseases. *American Journal of Epidemiology* 150:747–755.

38. Ford, G.W., Doyle, L.W., Davis, N.M. & Callanan, C. (2000). Very low birthweight and growth into adolescence. *Archives of Pediatric and Adolescent Medicine* 154:778–784.

39. Hediger, M.L., Overpeck, M.D., Kuczmarski, R.J., McGlynn, A., Maurer, K.R. & Davis, W.W. (1998). Muscularity and fatness of infants and young children born small- or large-for-gestational age. *Pediatrics* 102: e60.

40. Yau, K-I.T. & Chang, M-H. (1993). Growth and body composition of

preterm, small-for-gestational-age infants at a postmenstrual age of 37–40 weeks. *Early Human Development* 33:117–131.

41. Larsson, B., Svardsudd, K., Welin, L., Wilhelmsen, L., Bjorntorp, P. & Tibblin, G. (1984). Abdominal adipose tissue distribution, obesity, and risk of cardiovascular disease and death: 13-year follow-up of participants in the study of men born in 1913. *British Medical Journal* 288:1401–4.

42. Law, C.M., Barker, D.J.P., Osmond, C. Fall, C.H.D. & Simmonds, S.J. (1992). Early growth and abdominal fatness in adult life. *Journal of Epidemiology and Community Health* 46:184–6.

43. Hediger, M.L., Scholl, T.O., Schall, J.I. & Cronk, C.E. (1995). One-year changes in weight and fatness in girls during late adolescence. *Pediatrics* 96:253–8.

44. Van Lenthe, F.J., van Mechelen, W., Kemper, H.C.G. & Twisk, J.W.R. (1998). Association of a central pattern of body fat with blood pressure and lipoproteins from adolescence into adulthood. *American Journal of Epidemiology* 147:686–693.

45. Haffner, S.M., Stern, M.P., Hazuda, H.P., et al. (1986). Upper-body and centralized adiposity in Mexican Americans and non-Hispanic whites: Relationship to body mass index and other behavioral and demographic variables. *International Journal of Obesity* 10:493–502.

46. Malina, R.M., Katzmarzyk, P.T. & Beunen, G. (1996). Birthweight and its relationship to size attained and relative fat distribution at 7 to 12 years of age. *Obesity Research* 4:385–390.

47. Barker, M., Robinson, S., Osmond, C. & Barker, D.J.P. (1997). Birthweight and body fat distribution in adolescent girls. *Archives of Diseases of Children* 77:381–3.

48. Meyer, F., Moisan, J., Marcoux, D. & Bouchard, C. (1990). Dietary and physical determinants of menarche. *Epidemiology* 1:377–381.

49. Frisch, R.E. & McArthur, J.W. (1974). Menstrual cycles: Fatness as a determinant of minimum weight for height necessary for their maintenance or onset. *Science* 185:949–950.

50. Cresswell, J.L., Egger, P., Fall, C.H.D., Osmond, C., Fraser, R.B. & Barker, D.J.P. (1997). Is the age of menopause determined in utero? *Early Human Development* 49:143–8.

51. Francois, I. & de Zegher, F. (1997). Adrenarche and fetal growth. *Pediatric Research* 41:440–442.

52. Kelsey, J.L., Gammon, M.D. & John, E.M. (1993). Reproductive factors and breast cancer. *Epidemiologic Reviews* 15:36–47.

53. Hunter, D.J. & Willett, W.C. (1993). Diet, body size, and breast cancer. *Epidemiologic Reviews* 15:110–132.
54. Cooper, G.S. & Sandler, D.P. (1997). Long-term effects of reproductive-age menstrual cycle patterns on peri- and postmenopausal fracture risk. *American Journal of Epidemiology* 145:804–9.
55. Johnell, O. & Nilsson, B.E. (1984). Lifestyle and bone mineral mass in perimenopausal women. *Calcified Tissue International* 36:354–6.
56. Fox, K.M., Magaziner, J., Sherwin, R., et al. (1993). Reproductive correlates of bone mass in elderly women. *Journal of Bone Mineral Research* 8:901–8.
57. Paganinini-Hill, A., Chao, A., Ross, R.K., et al. (1991). Exercise and other factors in the prevention of hip fracture: the Leisure World study. *Epidemiology* 2:16–25.
58. Warren, M.P., Brooks-Gunn, J., Fox, R.P., Lancelot, C., Newman, D. & Hamilton, W.G. (1991). Lack of bone accretion and amenorrhea: Evidence for a relative osteopenia in weight-bearing bones. *Journal of Clinical Endocrinology and Metabolism* 72:847–853.
59. Wyshak, G. (2000). Teenaged girls, carbonated beverage consumption, and bone fractures. *Archives of Pediatric and Adolescent Medicine* 154:610–613.
60. Ludwig, D.S., Pereira, M.A., Kroenke, C.H., Hilner, J.E., Van Horn, L., Slattery, M.L. & Jacobs, D.R. (1999). Dietary fiber, weight gain, and cardiovascular disease risk factors in young adults. *Journal of the American Medical Association* 282:1539–1546.
61. Strauss, R.S. (1999). Self-reported weight status and dieting in a cross-sectional sample of young adolescents. *Archives of Pediatrics and Adolescent Medicine* 153:741–7.
62. Pugliese, M.T., Lifshitz, F., Grad, G., Fort, P. & Marks-Katz, M. (1983). Fear of obesity: A cause of short stature and delayed puberty. *New England Journal of Medicine* 309:513–8.
63. Slemenda, C.W., Miller, J.Z., Hui, S.L., Reister, T.K. & Johnson, C.C. (1991). Role of physical activity in the development of skeletal mass in children. *Journal of Bone and Mineral Research* 6:1227–33.
64. Haliova, L. & Anderson, J.J.B. (1989). Lifetime calcium intake and physical activity habits: Independent and combined effects on the radial bone of healthy premenopausal women. *American Journal of Clinical Nutrition* 49:534–541.
65. McCulloch, R.C., Bailey, D.A., Houston, C.S. & Dodd, B.L. (1990).

Effects of physical activity, dietary calcium intake, and selected lifestyle factors on bone density in young women. *Canadian Medical Association Journal* 142:221–7.

66. Metz, J.A., Anderson, J.J.B. & Gallagher, P.N. (1993). Intakes of calcium, phosphorus, and protein, and physical activity level are related to radial bone mass in young adult women. *American Journal of Clinical Nutrition* 58:537–42.

67. Welten, D.C., Kemper, H.C.G., Post, G.B., et al. (1994). Weight-bearing activity during youth is a more important factor for peak bone mass than calcium intake. *Journal of Bone and Mineral Research* 9:1089–96.

68. Kriska, A.M., Sandler, R.B., Cauley, J.A., LaPorte, R.E., Hom, D.L. & Pambianco, G. (1988). The assessment of historical physical activity and its relation to adult bone parameters. *American Journal of Epidemiology* 127:1053–61.

69. Schoutens, A., Laurent, E. & Poortmans, J.R. (1989). Effects of inactivity and exercise on bone. *Sports Medicine* 7:71–81.

70. Snow-Harter, C. & Marcus, R. (1991). Exercise, bone mineral density, and osteoporosis. *Exercise and Sport Science Review* 19:351–88.

71. Telama, R., Yang, X., Laakso, L. & Viikari, J. (1997). Physical activity in childhood and adolescence as predictor of physical activity in young children. *American Journal of Preventive Medicine* 13:317–323.

72. Greendale, G.A., Barrett-Connor, E., Edelstein, S., Ingles, S. & Haile, R. (1995). Lifetime leisure exercise and osteoporosis: The Rancho Bernardo study. *American Journal of Epidemiology* 141:951–9.

73. Jaglal, S.B., Kreiger, N. & Darlington, G. (1993). Past and recent physical activity and risk of hip fracture. *American Journal of Epidemiology* 138:107–118.

74. Rico, H., Revilla, M., Villa, L.F., Gómez-Castresana, F. & Alvarez del Buergo, M. (1993). Body composition in postpubertal boy cyclists. *Journal of Sports Medicine and Physical Fitness* 33:278–81.

75. Smith, R. & Rutherford, O.M. (1993). Spine and total body bone mineral density and serum testosterone levels in male athletes. *European Journal of Applied Physiology* 67:330–4.

76. Nieman, D.C., Johanssen, L.M., Lee, J.W. & Arabatzis, K. (1990). Infectious episodes in runners before and after the Los Angeles marathon. *Journal of Sports Medicine and Physical Fitness* 30:316–328.

77. Frisch, R.E., Wyshak, G. & Vincent, L. (1980). Delayed menarche

and amenorrhea in ballet dancers. *New England Journal of Medicine* 303:17–19.

78. Warren, M.P., Brooks-Gunn, J., Hamilton, L.H., Warren, L.F. & Hamilton, W.G. (1986). Scoliosis and fractures in young ballet dancers. *New England Journal of Medicine* 314:1348–53.

79. Young, N., Formica, C. & Szmukler, G. (1994). Bone density at weight-bearing and non-weight-bearing sites in ballet dancers: The effects of exercise, hypogonadism, and body weight. *Journal of Clinical Endocrinology and Metabolism* 78:449–54.

80. Baer, J.T., Taper, L.J., Gwazdauskas, F.G., et al. (1992). Diet, hormonal, and metabolic factors affecting bone mineral density in adolescent amenorrheic and eumenorrheic female runners. *Journal of Sports Medicine and Physical Fitness* 32:51–8.

81. Jonnavithula, S., Warren, M.P., Foc, R.P. & Lazaro, M.I. (1993). Bone density is compromised in amenorrheic women despite return of menses: A 2-year study. *Obstetrics and Gynecology* 81:669–74.

82. Drinkwater, B.L., Bruemmer, B. & Chesnut, C.H. (1990). Menstrual history as a determinant of current bone density in young athletes. *Journal of the American Medical Association* 263:545–8.

83. Cann, C.E., Cavanagh, D.J., Schnurpfiel, K. & Martin, M.C. (1988). Menstrual history is the primary determinant of trabecular bone density in women. *Medicine and Science in Sports and Exercise Journal* 20 (Suppl 2):S59 Abs.

84. Cann, C.E., Martin, M.C. & Jaffee, R.B. (1985). Duration of amenorrhea affects rate of bone loss in women runners: Implications for therapy. *Medicine and Science in Sports and Exercise Journal* 17:214–9.

85. Shimokata, H., Muller, D.C. & Andres, R. (1989). Studies in the distribution of body fat. III. Effects of cigarette smoking. *Journal of the American Medical Association* 261:1169–1173.

Additional Studies of Interest

Anderson, J.J.B., Tylavsky, F.A., Lacey, J.M., Talmage, R.V. & Taft, T. (1987). Major factors influencing distal radial bone mass in college-age women. *Federation Proceedings* 46:632 (abstr).

Drinkwater, B.L., Nilson, K., Chesnut, C.H., Bremmer, W.J., Shainholtz, S. & Southworth, M.B. (1984). Bone mineral content of amenorrheic and eumenorrheic athletes. *New England Journal of Medicine* 311:277–281.

(1993). Female athlete triad risk for women. *Journal of the American Medical Association* 270:921–3.

Fischer, E.C., Nelson, M.E., Frontera, W.R., Turksoy, R.N. & Evans, W.J. (1986). Bone mineral content and levels of gonadotropins and estrogens in amenorrheic running women. *Journal of Clinical Endocrinology and Metabolism* 62:1232–6.

Haapasalo, H., Kannus, P., Sievänen, H., Heinonen, A., Oja, P. & Vuori, I. (1994). Long-term unilateral loading and bone mineral density and content in female squash players. *Calcified Tissue International* 54:249–55.

Hager, R.L., Tucker, L.A. & Seljaas, G.T. (1995). Aerobic fitness, blood lipids, and body fat in children. *American Journal of Public Health* 85:1702–6.

Lindberg, J.S., Fears, W.B., Hunt, M.M., Powell, M.R., Boll, D. & Wade, C.E. (1984). Exercise-induced amenorrhea and bone density. *Annals of Internal Medicine* 101:647–8.

Louis, O., Demeirleir, K., Kalender, W., et al. (1991). Low vertebral bone density values in young non-elite female runners. *International Journal of Sports Medicine* 12:214–7.

(1997). Monthly estimates of leisure-time physical inactivity—United States, 1994. *Morbidity and Mortality Weekly Report* 46:393–7.

Nelson, M.E., Fisher, E.C., Catsos, P.D., Meredith, C.N., Turksoy, R.N. & Evans, W.J. (1986). Diet and bone status in amenorrheic runners. *American Journal of Clinical Nutrition* 43:910–6.

Rencken, M.L., Chesnut, C.H. & Drinkwater, B.L. (1996). Bone density at multiple skeletal sites in amenorrheic athletes. *Journal of the American Medical Association* 276:238–240.

Slemenda, C.W. & Johnston, C.C. (1993). High-intensity activities in young women: Site specific bone mass effects among female figure skaters. *Bone Minerals* 20:125–32.

Snead, D.B., Stubbs, C.C., Weltman, J.Y. et al. (1992). Dietary patterns, eating behaviors, and bone mineral density in women runners. *American Journal of Clinical Nutrition* 56:705–11.

(1993). Toddler deaths resulting from ingestion of iron supplements—Los Angeles, 1992–1993. *Morbidity and Mortality Weekly Report* 42:111–3.

Tofler, I.R., Stryer, B.K., Micheli, L.J. & Herman, L.R. (1996). Physical and emotional problems of elite female gymnasts. *New England Journal of Medicine* 335:281–3.

INDEX

Index

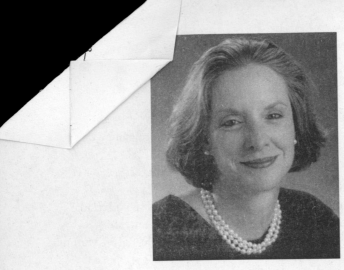

ABOUT THE AUTHORS

BARBARA LUKE, Sc.D., M.P.H., R.D., has an undergraduate degree in nursing from Columbia University, a master's degree in foods and nutrition from New York University and another in population studies from Columbia University, and a doctoral degree in maternal and child health from Johns Hopkins University. She has focused her career on prenatal nutrition and women's health. Her work has included clinical practice, research and teaching, public speaking to both professional and lay audiences, nationally and internationally, and publishing.

In addition to more than three dozen original research papers, numerous reviews, abstracts, and invited chapters, Dr. Luke is also the author or editor of fourteen books, including *Maternal Nutrition, Clinical Maternal-Fetal Nutrition, Multiple Pregnacy: Epidemiology, Gestation, and Perinatal Outcome, Every Pregnant Woman's Guide to Preventing Premature Birth, Good Bones: The Complete Guide to Building and Maintaining the Healthiest Bones,* and *When You're Expecting Twins, Triplets, or Quads.*

Her primary research interests include work and pregnancy, multiple births, and healthcare costs. Dr. Luke is Professor and Director, Division of Health Services Research, Department of Obstetrics and Gynecology, University of Michigan Medical School.

TAMARA EBERLEIN, an award-winning journalist, has published hundreds of articles on pregnancy, parenting, and health in national and international magazines. She is also the author of *Sleep: How to Teach Your Child to Sleep Like a Baby* and *Whining: Tactics for Taming Demanding Behavior.* Her previous collaboration with Dr. Barbara Luke, *When You're Expecting Twins, Triplets, or Quads,* has been hailed as the "bible of pregnancy books" for expectant mothers of multiples.